Discovering
Homeopathy
Medicine for the 21st Century

Discovering Homeopathy

Medicine for the 21st Century

Dana Ullman

North Atlantic Books
Berkeley, California

Publisher's address:
North Atlantic Books
2800 Woolsey Street
Berkeley, CA 94705

Cover art © Alex Grey, 1989 from the last panel of a
triptych entitled "Journey of the Wounded Healer."
Cover and book design by Paula Morrison
Typeset by Classic Typography

Discovering Homeopathy: Medicine for the 21st Century is sponsored by the
Society for the Study of Native Arts and Sciences, a nonprofit educational
corporation whose goals are to develop an ecological and crosscultural perspective linking various scientific, social, and artistic fields; to nurture a holistic
view of arts, sciences, humanities, and healing; and to publish and distribute
literature on the relationship of mind, body, and nature.

Library of Congress Cataloging-in-Publication Data

Ullman, Dana.
    Discovering Homeopathy : medicine for the 21 century.

    Bibliography: p.
    Includes index.
    1. Homeopathy.   I. Title. [DNLM: 1. Homeopathy.
WB 930 U41h]
RX71.U46   1988   615.5'32   87-28149
ISBN 1-55643-108-2

Contents

Foreword ix

Acknowledgments xi

Introduction to the 1991 Edition xiii

Introduction: Health, Illness, and Medicine
in the 21st Century xxiii
    Diseases of the 21st Century
    The Role of Homeopathy in the 21st Century
    Assumptions About Contemporary and
        21st-Century Medicine
    Notes

Part I: The Science and Art of Homeopathic Medicine

Chapter 1: A Modern Understanding of
Homeopathic Medicine 3
    Symptoms as Defenses
    Homeopathy's Basic Principle: The Law of Similars
    The Importance of Individualization
    The Use of Small Doses
    Understanding the Healing Process
    Homeopathic Typologies: The Bodymind Personalties
    Unconventional Approaches of Homeopathy
    The Limitations and Risks of Homeopathic Medicine
    Summary and Conclusion
    Notes

Chapter 2: A Condensed History of Homeopathy 33
    The Opposition to Homeopathy
    The Rise of Homeopathy
    The Fall of Homeopathy
    The Present Status of Homeopathy
    Notes

Chapter 3: Homeopathic Research:
Scientific Verification of Homeopathic Medicine 55
    The Empirical Evidence
    Clinical Evidence
    Clinical Trials on Animals
    Laboratory Evidence
    Implications of Homeopathic Research
    Notes

Part II: The Scope of Homeopathic Practice

Chapter 4: Pregnancy and Labor:
Getting Off to a Good Start 73
    Homeopathic Medicines in Pregnancy
    Homeopathic Medicines During Labor
    The Homeopathic Treatment of Mother and Infant
    Notes

Chapter 5: Pediatrics: Don't Drug Our Kids—
Give Them Homeopathics 91
    Medical Child Abuse
    The Homeopathic Alternative to Aspirin in Fevers
    The Homeopathic Treatment of Common Infant
        Health Problems: Teething, Colic, and Eczema
    The Homeopathic Treatment of Childhood Conditions
    The Story of Eric: A Great Kid and a Terror
    Notes

Chapter 6: Women's Health:
Treating, Not Mistreating, a Woman's Body 107
    The Homeopathic Treatment of PMS and Cystitis
    The Homeopathic Treatment of Vaginal Infections
        and Chronic Problems
    The Homeopathic Treatment of Menopause
    Notes

Chapter 7: Infectious Disease:
Effective Alternatives to Antibiotics 119
    The Homeopathic and Ecological View
      of Infectious Disease
    Are Antibiotics Helpful in Ear and Throat Infections?
    The Homeopathic Treatment of Infectious Disease
    The Homeopathic Treatment of Viral Conditions
    The Homeopathic Perspective on
      and Treatment of AIDS
    In Conclusion
    Notes

Chapter 8: Allergic Conditions:
Beyond Symptomatic Relief 139
    Conventional Medical Treatment for Allergies
    The Homeopathic Treatment of Allergies
    The Homeopathic Treatment of Food Allergies
    Notes

Chapter 9: The Treatment of Chronic Disease:
The Homeopathic Alternative........................ 153
    The Homeopaths' Understanding of Chronic Disease
    The Homeopathic Treatment of Chronic Disease
    A Case of Undiagnosed Chronic Abdominal Pain
    Notes

Chapter 10: Sports Medicine:
Achieving Peak Performance and Healing
Injuries Faster with Homeopathic Medicines 173
    Homeopathy and Sports Medicine
    Notes

Chapter 11: Psychological Problems:
Treating Mind and Body 185
    Modern Psychiatric Care
    The Homeopathic Understanding of Mental Illness
    The Homeopathic Treatment of Psychological Problems
    Psychotherapy: Homeopathic Style
    Notes

Chapter 12: Homeopathy and Dentistry:
Keeps You Smiling 203
    Homeopathic Insights on the
        Controversy of Fluoridation
    Amalgam Fillings: The Controversy
    Homeopathic Medicines for Dental Problems
    Notes

Chapter 13: Collaborative Health Care:
A Model for the 21st Century 219
    Notes

Appendix: Update on the Homeopathic
Treatment of AIDS 227

Part III: Homeopathic Resources

How to Learn More About Homeopathy 236

Starting and Participating in a
Homeopathic Study Group 243

Sources of Homeopathic Books, Tapes,
and General Information 249
    Homeopathic Manufacturers
    Homeopathic Organizations
    Schools and Training Programs in North America
    Introductory and Self-Care Books
    Philosophy, Methodology, and Research
    Materia Medicas and Repertories
    History of Homeopathy

Finding a Homeopathic Practitioner 254

A Note of Prediction and Caution 256

Index 258

Foreword

There is a great need to understand homoeopathy* in the light of modern science and to integrate it within a comprehensive health care system.

This book by Dana Ullman brings a modern freshness and insight into homoeopathy, which will go a long way to meeting these needs as described.

Textbooks in homoeopathy are a cause of great frustration. Many are more than 100 years old, few are less than 20 years old. Most of these make homoeopathy seem merely to be a 19th-century healing art. They cannot by virtue of antiquity or prejudice come to terms with 20th-century medical discoveries or insights into the disorders and sufferings of mankind.

But 20th-century people are now very sophisticated and demand information on homoeopathy in comprehensible language and with reference, where applicable, to modern research.

There is a need for a textbook which can be read by advocate or skeptic alike and which will allow a reasonable assessment of homoeopathy to be made. Such a textbook must be written without the necessity for special pleading or flights into quasi-mystical belief systems. There is a need for a book to set forth homoeopathy as a system of medicine for young, middle-aged, or elderly persons to use as a reference point in anticipation of, or during the suffering of, ill health.

It is therefore a pleasure to recommend this book, which will probably become a major introductory book on the subject of homoeopathy. Besides describing the principles of homoeopathy, it covers the history, the research, and the various applications

---

*Originally spelled "homoeopathy" and still spelled this way by many, "homeopathy" is a modern spelling that is widely used in the United States and beginning to be used in other countries.

of homoeopathy in clinical practice. It therefore deals with obstetric conditions, gynaecological disorders, paediatric complaints, infectious diseases, allergies, chronic illnesses, sports injuries, mental illness, and dental disease.

In summary, this book does not set out to be a self-care manual. Instead, it informs the reader of the usefulness of homoeopathy in a wide variety of acute and chronic complaints. Benefit only can accrue from reading it.

Ronald Davey
Physician to Her Majesty
Queen Elizabeth II

Acknowledgments

I have been honored to have had so many fine friends and colleagues give me no-nonsense feedback on my writings.

Randall Neustaedter, C.A.; Bernardo Merizalde, M.D.; and Stephen Cummings, F.N.P., have been particularly helpful by reviewing significant portions of the book.

The following friends and colleagues reviewed at least a portion of the book and provided some valuable information that has been incorporated into it: Jacqueline Wilson, M.D.; Bill Shevin, M.D.; Richard Moskowitz, M.D.; Alan Trachtenberg, M.D.; Linda Johnston, M.D.; Harris Coulter, Ph.D.; Jeffrey Gould, M.D., M.P.H.; Ananda Zaren, R.N.; Julian Winston; Harvey Powelson, M.D.; George Baldwin, D.D.S.; Richard Fischer, D.D.S.; Philip Parsons, D.D.S.; Janet Zand, C.A., N.D.; Marcel Simons, M.D.; Jacques Imbrechts, M.D.; Sandra Chase, M.D.; Jonathan Shore, M.D.; Jeff Baker, N.D.; John George, M.D.; Ben Hole, M.D.; Steve Subotnick, D.P.M.; Bart Flick, M.D.; Penelope Roberts, D.C.; Michael Quinn, R.Ph.; Gregory Manteuffel, M.D.; Sandra McLanahan, M.D.; Dean Ornish, M.D.; Ernest Callenbach; Beverly Chapman; Steve Waldstein; Shandor Weiss, N.D.; Andy Hendrickson; and Elizabeth Hallett.

My colleagues in the United Kingdom have been close to me despite the physical distance between us. David Taylor Reilly, M.B., M.R.C.P.; Morag Taylor; Peter Fisher, M.B., M.R.C.P.; and Francis Treuherz have helped make some important contributions to this book and have helped me feel connected to the international community of homeopaths.

I thank the Planetree Resource Center in San Francisco, which is a veritable treasure house of medical books, journals, and newsletters. The very existence of Planetree was invaluable in helping me get access to up-to-date medical information.

Paula Morrison designed the front cover, and Chris Mole

xi

drew the innovative caduceus for it. Their fine work deserves recognition.

Paul Weisser did the final copy-edit, and I sincerely thank him for making certain that I dotted my *i*'s and crossed my *t*'s.

Some friends whose own work and lives have inspired me include: Steven Schmidt; Marc Lappé, Ph.D.; Jack Warren Salmon, Ph.D.; Stephen Rosenblatt, Ph.D., C.A.; Kathy Rosenblatt, C.A.; Fritjof Capra, Ph.D.; Mark Satin; Denny Thompson; Betsy Boardman; Nalini Chilkov; and Allan Solares. I thank them dearly.

A particular thanks to Patricia Fisher for her special support, and to David Hoskinson for the occasional kick in the pants.

Richard Grossinger, my editor, publisher, and friend, deserves special credit for lending his wisdom to the editing process and for his midwifery skills in helping to give birth to this book.

Robert Bruce Moody and Jocelyn Elder-Gray are my assistants who have made and continue to make everything a lot easier. Their never-ending enthusiasm for life and good work has helped make the day-to-day sweat of working together joyful and productive.

My special appreciation goes to my father, Sanford Ullman, whose medical background in pediatrics and allergies was invaluable in his editing of several chapters of this book and whose fatherly guidance, support, and love have been an enduring and enriching lifeline to me.

Introduction to the 1991 Edition

For two centuries homeopathy has attracted the support and encouragement of royalty, the educated elite, and leading artists. It was thus no surprise that the most expensive painting ever sold was that of a portrait of a homeopath, Dr. Gachet, drawn by his personal friend and patient, Vincent Van Gogh. Although homeopaths may advocate the use of exceedingly small doses of medicines, people greatly value their homeopaths and the doses they prescribe. In this case, the portrait of Dr. Gachet sold for $82.5 million.

This portrait did not sell for this astronomical amount because it was of a homeopath, though one can wonder if its value will increase as homeopathy continues to gain in popularity.

And indeed, homeopathy's popularity is growing. According to a recent survey, 32% of the French public have used homeopathic medicines.[1] In another survey an astounding 59% of French family practice physicians stated that they were interested or open to homeopathy, and an impressive 32% stated that they had already incorporated homeopathy into their practice.[2]

According to a survey in the *British Medical Journal,* 42% of British physicians refer patients to homeopathic physicians.[3] Another survey in England indicated that 11% of the population had tried homeopathy, and 80% expressed satisfaction with the treatment, while only 7% were dissatisfied.[4] Homeopathy is the fastest growing form of alternative medicine in Scotland. In 1985, 23% of the

Scottish public said they would seriously consider seeking homeopathic care, while 40% of the population would have done so in 1989.[5]

Despite homeopathy's popularity throughout Europe, it is even more popular in India. There are over 100 four- and five-year homeopathic medical colleges, and homeopathy continues to receive increasing governmental support. Additional evidence of homeopathy's integration into the mainstream comes from the 1987 establishment in six New Delhi police stations of drug de-tox units in which homeopathy was the primary treatment. A 30-month study of 200 patients showed impressive results.[6]

One might wonder if and when these other countries will send Peace Corps teams of homeopaths to the United States.

New Research/New Controversies

Since this book was first published in 1988, new research has tended to confirm the value of the homeopathic medicine and has also created new controversies.

The most significant occurred in mid-1988 when Dr. Jacques Benveniste, one of the leading allergists in Europe, led a group of scientists in a series of experiments which were ultimately published in *Nature*,[7] perhaps the most respected scientific journal in the world. Dr. Benveniste's research was confirmed by scientists at three other universities: University of Toronto, University of Milano, and Hebrew University.

Dr. Benveniste is a highly respected scientist and physician. He has authored 13 previous articles, each of which has been cited in over 100 research articles. He considers his research using microdoses to be as good as any of his other research.

The experiment itself was quite technical. Basically, the experimenters used exceedingly small doses of an antibody to see if it would affect basophils, a type of white blood cell that reacts to allergens. The experimenters diluted doses of the antibody from 1:10 up to 120 times. Although such minute doses are typically used by homeopaths in daily practice, skeptics assume that these microdoses could not possibly have any biological action or clinical effect.

Although the experimenters conducted their experiment 70 times, the editor of *Nature*, John Maddox, published a disclaimer next to the article questioning the authenticity of the experiments' results. Maddox also asserted that he would not publish the article unless Benveniste permitted an investigative team to come to his laboratory at the University of Paris South to try to replicate the experiment. Because Benveniste felt he had nothing to hide, he encouraged this challenge, even though Maddox's request was unprecedented in science.

Rather than assembling peer scientists, Maddox put together an investigative team including magician James "The Amazing" Randi and fraud expert Walter Stewart.

This team asked Benveniste and colleagues to replicate the experiment seven times. The first three times were not in a "blind" fashion. In other words, the experimenter who looked through the microscope to count the number of basophils knew when she was reading those treated with the microdoses and when she was reading those treated with the placebo. Although these experiments showed the effect from the microdoses, everybody considered these results invalid because of the inherent bias in the experiment. The experimenters had never before done their tests in this unscientific fashion but complied with the investigative team's request so that they would not seem uncooperative.

In the next experiment, the experimenter was "blinded." She did not know which slides had been treated with the microdoses and which received the placebo. Much to the surprise of the skeptics, the experiment again showed significant differences between the effect of the microdose and the placebo. The skeptics, however, determined that this test was also invalid. Instead, they now asserted that the person looking through the microscope be blinded AND the person who was dropping the microdoses onto the slides be blinded from knowing if microdoses or placebos were used.

Although this extra blinding adds further protection from potential bias, the simple blinding of the person reading the microscope is more than adequate to evaluate the objective results of the experiment.

When the next three tests were conducted, however, the cells treated with the microdoses were not different from those given a placebo. The skeptics immediately declared that the microdoses were proven to be ineffective,[8] and virtually every major newspaper and news magazine, including *Time* and *Newsweek*, echoed this "proof."

The media did highlight the unusual nature of the investigative team, noting that none were experts in allergy or immunology. This investigative team was thus not knowledgeable of the simple fact that allergological and immunological experiments of this sort very rarely achieve 100% positive results. In fact, it is common for scientists to achieve positive results 30–50% of the time and be considered significant. If anyone on the investigative team had been better informed about this issue, the group would have known that conducting simply three trials was inadequate.

Worse still, not a single media source mentioned the fact that one of the four experiments showed that the microdoses acted.

To add insult to injury, when Benveniste recently conducted even more strictly controlled trials of this experiment, he submitted his research to *Nature* and to *Science,* but neither was willing to publish it. In an effort to further silence healthy scientific dialog on this important subject, Benveniste's employer at the French National Institute for Scientific Research in Medicine has asked him to stop conducting research into microdose effects.

Science is not well served by stopping the investigation of controversial topics. Yet skeptics feel that science has disproved the possible biological activity of homeopathic microdoses and that the subject is now closed.

The same skeptics, however, seem to have ignored the fact that Benveniste's experiment was not the first or the last study on homeopathy (see Chapter 3 for details about research previous to 1988). And new research has lent further support to the potency of homeopathic microdoses.

New Clinical Research

In a double-blind experiment of patients with influenza almost twice as many given a homeopathic medicine recovered from the flu within 48 hours (as compared with those patients given a placebo). This experiment was conducted on 487 people who were referred for treatment by 149 different physicians. The prestigious journal *The Lancet* was so impressed by this study that they reported not only on its results but on how well it was conducted.[9]

What was additionally important about this study was the fact that only one medicine was used, and thus no individualization of symptoms was attempted. Since homeopaths commonly feel that results would be even better with such individualization, getting good results with only one medicine is impressive. The medicine used was *Anas barbariae hepatica cordis* 200c (commonly marketed as *Oscillococcinum*).

The "200c" written after this medicine indicates that it was diluted 1:100 200 times, which is considerably more dilute than the medicine used in the Benveniste experiment.

Another experiment worthy of mention was one published in the *British Medical Journal* which described research on the treatment of patients with a rheumatological condition called fibrositis (also called primary fibromyalgia).[10]

This experiment utilized the most sophisticated form of experimental design called "double-blind and cross-over." "Double-blind" means that neither the experimenter nor the subject know who received the "real" medicine and who received the placebo. "Cross-over" means that during the first half of the experiment half of the subjects are given a placebo, while the other half are given the "real" medicine; then during the second half, those who began with the placebo get the "real" medicine and those who began with the "real" medicine get the placebo.

What makes this type of study credible is that it doesn't simply compare one patient with another; it compares a patient under one treatment with that same patient under another treatment.

Although this experiment gave every patient the same medicine, the experimenters only admitted 42% of fibrositis patients interviewed because only these people had symptoms that fit the homeopathic symptomology of the medicine used, *Rhus tox* (poison ivy). This study showed that the homeopathic medicine *Rhus tox* 6c was successful in reducing the number and amount of painful spots shortly after patients took this medicine.

Another double-blind experiment was performed on 61 people with varicose veins.[11] Conducted in Germany, this study used a combination of eight homeopathic medicines: *Meliotus* (sweet clover) 1x, *Aesculus* (horse chestnut) 1x, *Carduus marianus* (St. Mary's thistle) 1x, *Arnica* tincture (mountain daisy), *Lycopodium* (club moss) 4x, *Lachesis* (venom of the bushmaster) 4x, and *Rutin* 1x. The subjects of the experiment were given three doses daily for 24 days.

This study measured various objective and subjective symptoms of the patients. The results showed an astounding difference between those patients given the homeopathic medicines and those given the placebo. Those given the homeopathic medicines improved by 44%, while those given the placebo deteriorated 18%.

In another article published in *Thorax* the case of a 59-year-old man was described.[12] This patient had a type of lung cancer in which the average length of survival if left untreated is six to 17 weeks from the time of diagnosis. However, as the result of homeopathic treatment and the use of the herb mistletoe (Iscador), this patient lived five years seven months after diagnosis.

A single successful case is never "proof" of a specific treatment; however, cases such as this in which the predicted length of survival is significantly improved provide additional evidence for a therapy. And people who get homeopathic care often share similar stories of lengthened life, improvement in health, and just feeling better.

Learning from History

Although homeopathy has been a relatively popular and respected medical practice throughout the world, it has often been attacked by conventional physicians and their organizations. Their attacks on homeopathy and against specific homeopaths, however, have often led to increased support for this medical underdog (see Chapter 2 on "The History of Homeopathy" for more details).

A classic and recent example of this is the case of Dr. George Guess, a board certified family practice physician in North Carolina, who had his medical license revoked by the North Carolina medical board for committing the heinous crime of practicing homeopathy. Although no patient complained, the medical board considered Dr. Guess' practice to be "not in accordance with community standards of medicine."

Dr Guess appealed the medical board's decision to the Superior Court, and he won. In support of Dr. Guess' right to practice homeopathy, the court determined that the medical board's action was "arbitrary and capricious." The board then appealed this decision to the North Carolina Board of Appeals which ultimately agreed with the Superior Court, stating that the medical board acted improperly, though the court determined that their action was not "arbitrary and capricious."

Then, in 1990, the medical board appealed this decision to the North Carolina Supreme Court which overturned both lower courts and determined that the medical board could determine if physicians were not practicing according to "acceptable and prevailing" standards.[13]

The Supreme Court asserted that the popularity of homeopathic medicine in any other state or country was irrelevant, thus affirming that its status as a prevailing medical practice in North Carolina was the only appropriate measure of its acceptability. The Court also stipulated that whatever research that has proved or disproved homeopathy was not relevant, since the Court was only considering homeopathy's present prevalence in the state. Since very few physicians practiced homeopathy there at the time, the Court said that the medical board could determine that homeopathy was not acceptable.*

The North Carolina's Supreme Court action institutionalized provincialism. Homeopathy's popularity, research, and history were ignored.

And yet, from the beginning of this court case, Dr. Guess' practice has never been busier. The press in the case has been consistently sympathetic to homeopathy and to Dr. Guess. As has often been the case in history, attacks against homeopathy and homeopaths lead to its increasing popularity.

George Bernard Shaw once said, "One thing that we learn from history is that we don't learn from history." It is indeed sad that in this land of freedom some people seek to "protect" others from making their own decisions in health care. Hopefully as we approach the 21st century and as more and more countries experience "glasnost" and "perestroika," America will re-commit itself to real freedom and real democracy. In this process we will also begin to commit ourselves to real healing.

---

*As of this writing, the ACLU has joined Dr. Guess' case in efforts to defend freedom of choice in health care. The ACLU has long championed the constitutional rights of individuals, though this is their first effort to defend the freedom to choose unorthodox medical care.

Addendum

Just as we went to press on this new edition, a survey of homeopathic research appeared in the *British Medical Journal**. This
reviewed 107 controlled clinical trials performed between 1966 and
1990 in which homeopathic medicines were used. Of the 105 experiments with interpretable results, 81 showed positive results from
homeopathic medicines, while 24 found no benefit from them.

Despite these impressive results, the authors note that many
of the experiments had methodological problems. Of the 107 studies,
64 had fewer than 25 patients per control group, 39 were not ran-
domly chosen to receive either the treatment or the placebo, and
40 did not have a treatment outcome that was sensible and well
described.

Still, the vast majority of the best studies showed the value of
the homeopathic medicines. Of the 16 best studies done, 14 showed
positive effects of homeopathic medicines. Elsewhere in this book,
reference is made to several of these studies, including those which
showed the successful treatment of influenza (earlier in this chapter), childbirth (p. 84), and hay fever (p. 146).

Other studies that showed the value of homeopathic medicines
include their use in the treatment of migraine headaches, ankle
sprains, dry cough, post-operative infections, and symptoms after
abdominal surgery. There were additional studies showing positive
results in the treatment of influenza and hay fever.

Many people were not previously familiar with these studies
because a large portion of them were published in French or German medical and scientific journals.

Of the various studies, 13 of the 19 trials showed successful
treatment of respiratory infections, 6 of 7 trials showed positive
results in treating other infections, 5 of 7 trials showed improvement in diseases of the digestive system, 5 of 5 showed successful
treatment of hay fever, 5 of 7 showed faster recovery after abdominal surgery, 4 of 6 promoted healing in treating rheumatological dis-

---

*Kleijnen, J., Knipschild, P., and Gerben ter Riet, "Clinical Trials of
Homoeopathy," *British Medical Journal*, 302 (February 9, 1991): 316–323.

ease, 18 of 20 showed benefit in addressing pain or trauma, 8 of 10 showed efficacy in relieving mental or psychological problems, and 13 of 15 availed various diagnoses.

The authors, who are experts in analyzing clinical research and are not homeopathic physicians, concluded that their survey indicates that there is a legitimate case for further evaluation of homeopathy. Further, they specifically state that there is now sufficient evidence for using homeopathic medicine as a regular treatment for certain conditions.

This survey was financed by a grant from the Dutch Ministry of Welfare, Public Health, and Cultural Affairs, which explains why the article begins with a reference to Dutch physicians, 45% of whom think that homeopathic medicines are efficacious in treating upper respiratory tract infections or hay fever.

Notes

1.Bouchayer, "Alternative Medicines: A General Approach to the French Situation," *Complementary Medical Research*, 4 (May, 1990): 4–8.

2. Poll I.F.O.P., February, 1989. "Medecines douches: La revanche de l'homeopathie," *Le Nouvel Observateur*, April 12, 1985, 36–41.

3. Wharton, Richard, and George Lewith, "Complementary Medicine and the General Practitioner," *British Medicine Journal*, 292 (June 7, 1986): 1498–1500.

4. "Take a Little of What Ails You," *The Times*, November 13, 1989.

5. *Ibid.*

6. "National Congress on Homoeopathy and Drug Abuse," New Delhi, India, Sponsored by the Foundation for Medical Research and Education and the Delhi Police Foundation for Correction, Dedication and Rehabilitation, March 16–18, 1990.

7. Davenas, E., *et al.*, "Human Basophil Degranulation Triggered by Very Dilute Antiserum Against AgE," *Nature*, 333 (June 30, 1988): 816–818.

8. Maddox, J., Randi, J., and W. Stewart, "'High-dilution' Experiments a Delusion," *Nature*, 334 (July 28, 1988): 443–447.

9. Ferley, J. P., Zmirou, D., D'Adhemar, D., and F. Balducci, "A Controlled Evaluation of a Homeopathic Preparation in the Treatment of Influenza-like Syndromes," *British Journal of Clinical Pharmacology*, 1989, 299 (March, 1989): 365–366.

10. Fisher, P., Greenwood, A., Huskisson, E. C., Turner, P., and P. Belon. "Effect of Homoeopathic Treatment on Fibrositis (primary fibromyalgia)," *British Medical Journal.* 229 (August 5, 1989): 365–366.

11. Ernst, E., Saradeth, T., and K. L. Resch, "Complementary Treatment of Varicose Veins: A Randomised, Placebo-controlled, Double-blind Trial," *Phlebology,* 5 (1990): 157–163.

12. Bradley, G. W. and A. Clover, "Apparent Response of Small Cell Lung Cancer to an Extract of Mistletoe and Homeopathic Treatment," *Thorax,* 44 (1989): 1047–1048.

13. Guess v. North Carolina Board of Medical Examiners, North Carolina Supreme Court, July 28, 1990.

Introduction

Health, Illness, and Medicine in the 21st Century

When Elvis Presley died, coroners discovered nine different drugs in his body. In an effort to prevent embarrassment, one of his physicians sought to reassure the public that there were "sound, rational medical reasons" for all nine drugs. This reassurance may have protected Elvis from embarrassment, but it ultimately indicted conventional medicine for its presumption that there could ever be "sound, rational medical reasons" for giving nine different drugs to an individual at one time.

As valuable as conventional medicine is, it also has its limitations and problems. Because conventional drugs are usually prescribed for their individual capacities to act upon specific parts of the body, it follows that several different drugs might be prescribed to treat the various symptoms of one individual. And, of course, it then follows that additional drugs would be needed to control the side effects of one or more of the other drugs being taken.

Homeopathic medicine offers an alternative. Instead of giving one medicine for a person's headache, another for his constipation, another for his irritability, and yet another to counteract the effects of one or more of the medicines, the homeopathic physician prescribes a single medicine at a time that will stimulate the person's immune and defense capacity and bring about an overall improvement in that person's health. The procedure by which the homeopath finds the precise individual substance is the very science and art of homeopathy.

Medicine is at its very best when it incorporates the scientific method and the art of healing. Homeopathic medicine embodies such a system. This does not mean that homeopathy is the be-all and end-all of healing. Though homeopathic medicine is a profound and powerful means to stimulate a person's healing processes, it complements other health and medical care. Sound nutrition, exercise, stress management, emotional and mental balance, and effective conventional medical care together comprise a comprehensive health care system that fulfills the varied needs of our complex society.

As we enter the 21st century, a new type of comprehensive health care will emerge, one in which various natural healing practices and conventional medical treatments play an integral role. It will emerge not only because people will realize that it is the rational alternative, but also because it is necessary for physical, mental, and spiritual health.

Diseases of the 21st Century

Diseases of the 21st century will inevitably be different from those of the 20th century, just as our present illnesses have been quite different from those of the 19th century. Although our health is improving in many ways and we are living longer than in previous decades, new diseases and conditions threaten the quality of our lives. We have already observed some significant changes in the 1980s that portend what health problems lie ahead in the 21st century:

- Diseases of the immune system, not just AIDS but various conditions of a deficient or overactive immune system, have reached epidemic proportions.*
- The number of people suffering from viral conditions that are incurable with conventional therapies is increasing, and the number of newly defined viral conditions, such as the

---

*References to each of the trends mentioned here are provided in forthcoming chapters.

Epstein-Barr virus and cytomegaloviruses, is also increasing significantly.

- More and more bacterial infections are becoming resistant to commonly used antibiotics and are requiring stronger and stronger antibiotics, which also are not always successful in curing the infections.
- Allergies to foods, to common substances, and to new chemicals are becoming more and more prevalent.
- Chronic disability is affecting people more frequently at younger and younger ages.
- Mental disease is affecting more and more people.

In addition to these various trends, one of the more significant facts that will affect the future of health care is that a larger percentage of the population will be over 65 years old. According to projections by the U.S. Bureau of Census, the size of the American population over 65 in 1985 will have doubled by 2030.[1]

Futurists generally assume that 21st-century medicine will include new and more powerful drugs and various innovative technological interventions. However, futurists tend to ignore the serious problems presently arising from conventional medications. According to 1986 statistics, the average American receives 7.5 prescriptions a year.[2] This is a particularly frightening number because we all know people who have not been prescribed *any* medications in the past year, which means that someone else is getting *their* 7.5 drugs. Since most drugs have side effects, some of which are quite serious, and since the sick person is often prescribed several drugs at the same time, any of which may have even greater potential for side effects, it is no wonder that 50 percent of the time people do not even get their drug prescriptions filled. Additionally, various studies have indicated that 25 to 90 percent of the time patients make errors in administering the medicines.[3] Despite the respect that people generally have for present-day physicians, there does not seem to be equal confidence in the treatments they prescribe.

Most futurists who have written about health care in the 21st century tend to ignore these serious problems. They discuss new ways to use computers, scanners, and other technologies and only rarely describe many of the natural therapies that have been used for centuries and that have become increasingly popular in the 1970s and 1980s.

In contrast to most other futurists, Clement Bezold, Rick Carlson, and Jonathan Peck—in their book *The Future of Work and Health*—have predicted that 21st-century medicine will have a high-tech component but an equally strong "high-touch" component.[4] As well as new technological diagnostic and therapeutic measures, there will be significantly greater reliance on self-care practices; wellness programs; therapeutic, nutritional, and fitness regimens; and other alternative healing practices. The authors also note that science has already begun to recognize and will soon more fully integrate concepts about how one's psychological state affects various physiological processes. Wedding the medical specialties of psychiatry, neurology, and internal medicine, psychoneuroimmunology is fast becoming the formally acknowledged field of scientific inquiry into the relationship between mind and body.[5] Its practitioners attempt to understand and prevent disease in a holistic, scientific fashion and are presently developing methods that accelerate recovery and obtain higher states of health.

Bezold, Carlson, and Peck also predict that enlarged concepts of health will open science and medicine to various spiritual practices in health and healing. Meditation will be valued for its capacity to induce states of relaxation and heightened awareness. Laying on of hands by people of various religious orientations will become more prominent. And faith healing, which has always been popular, will attract scientific and medical sanction.

It is difficult to imagine 21st-century medicine without a high-touch component. Not only will reliance on technological medicine be too costly, but high-tech medicine has generally been very ineffective in treating a large number of common acute and chronic ailments. Although cures for various conditions have always seemed to be "just around the corner," the fact of the matter is that real cures from the use of conventional medical treatments have remained elusive. For so many conditions, conventional physicians do not claim to even "cure" but only to "manage" them. Conventional medical therapies may have significantly reduced the health-damaging effects of acute infectious diseases and have provided heroic interventions in dealing with a panoply of medical emergencies; and yet, the family physician and the medical specialist cannot effectively treat most chronic symptoms, syndromes, and diseases from which large numbers of people suffer. Since chronic afflictions will probably be even more prevalent than they are now as the median age of the population increases, therapeutic methods that not only manage or control symptoms but that effectively cure them must be the goal of medicine and science.

There are also a significant number of people today whose diagnosis eludes medical professionals. Often described as having a "nonspecific" or "undifferentiated" illness, these people are not often given effective treatment with conventional therapies. Clearly, alternative and complementary diagnostic and therapeutic approaches are necessary to provide effective health care. Homeopathic medicine offers this potential. Homeopathy will often complement orthodox medical care, and at other times it will replace it. Specifics of how homeopathy has been and is being utilized to treat modern-day and future health problems are discussed in later chapters of this book. By providing a diagnostic system that assesses the whole organism rather than simply its parts, and by being a therapeutic system that works by stimulating a person's own immune and defense system rather than by simply controlling or suppressing symptoms, homeopathy will inevitably become an integral part of health care in the United States.

The Role of Homeopathy in the 21st Century

Most Americans today know little or nothing about homeopathic medicine, despite the fact that 15 percent of American physicians at the turn of the century considered themselves to be homeopaths,[6] and despite the fact that homeopathy is so popular throughout the world today.[7] Homeopathic medicine is a natural pharmaceutical system that utilizes microdoses of substances from the plant, mineral, or animal kingdom to arouse a person's natural healing response. Homeopathy is a sophisticated method of individualizing small doses of medicines in order to initiate that healing response. Unlike conventional drugs, which act primarily by having direct effects upon physiological processes related to a person's symptoms, homeopathic medicines are thought to work by stimulating the person's immune and defense system, which raises his or her overall level of health, thereby enabling him or her to reestablish health and prevent disease.

Homeopathy, of course, cannot cure everything or everybody, but it does offer the real possibility of cure for various deep-seated acute, chronic, and hereditary diseases. Some research (which will be discussed in other chapters) has begun to verify this claim, though certainly more scientific investigation is necessary to determine how effective homeopathy is and how to make it even more effective.

As scientists and the general public develop greater understanding and respect for the body's immune system, homeopathy will gain in popularity as a primary pharmacological means to stimulate immune response. Those conventional medical therapies that primarily treat and suppress symptoms will be accepted for their valuable role in health care, but not necessarily as a first course of treatment.*

As important as antibiotics are in treating bacterial infections, a growing number of these infections are becoming resistant to known antibiotics. Medical observers generally predict that this trend will continue into the 21st century. New and stronger antibiotics will inevitably be developed, but alternative pharmacological means must play an important role in the control and cure of infectious diseases.

Homeopathic medicines are also likely to become the treat-

---

*Reference to "conventional medicine" and "conventional medical treatment" applies to medical care commonly practiced in the mid-1980s. It is a bit odd to utilize this term, since what is conventional today may be considered quackery tomorrow and what is considered quackery today may become part of conventional medicine tomorrow. A similar semantic dilemma exists for the term "alternative health care," which is rapidly becoming an inappropriate term because it is not an "alternative" to many people. In fact, what may be termed "alternative medicine" is probably being used by more people in the world than what is termed "conventional medicine." In recognition of these problems, this book will still utilize the terms "conventional medicine" and "alternative medicine" in accordance with their definitions in the mid-1980s.

ment of choice in viral conditions. Conventional medicine today offers little curative care for those people suffering from serious viral infections or even, for that matter, common mild viruses. In his seminal book *The Mirage of Health,* Pulitzer Prize-winning microbiologist René Dubos expresses concern about conventional medicine's ability to deal with various types of infection, and doubts if conventional medicine will be effective in its treatment of these conditions until a shift in thinking and practice takes place within medicine. "One might assume," he writes, "that the persistence of microbial disease is merely a temporary situation, a problem soon to be solved by the discovery of new and more powerful drugs. In reality, there are limitations inherent in drug therapy even under the most favorable conditions. Some of these limitations are technical and cannot be discussed here. Others are more fundamental in character, having their basis in the very philosophy of disease control."[8]

Homeopathy offers a different philosophy, since its medicines are not simply intended to be antibacterial or antiviral but to stimulate the person's overall resistance to infection. Homeopathic medicines strengthen the organism so that it is more capable of defending itself, and do so without producing the side effects commonly experienced with antibiotics. Such treatment provides a more ecological approach to curing infectious disease, since it aids the body's natural homeostasis without suppressing the organism's inherent self-protective responses.

Homeopathy actually became popular in the United States and Europe in the first place because of its successes in treating the various infectious epidemic diseases that were rampant in the 19th century.[9] I predict that homeopathic medicines will be an integral part of the medical treatment of infectious conditions in the future. Antibiotics will, no doubt, still be commonly prescribed, but they will be used significantly less often than they are today.

Since homeopathic medicines are known to be considerably safer than conventional drugs, their use in the 21st century will sharply reduce the amount of iatrogenic (doctor-induced) disease. One 1981 study that evaluated the reasons for admission to a respected university hospital in Boston revealed that an astonishing 36 percent of the patients were admitted for iatrogenic conditions.[10]

Homeopathy will provide a distinct resolution of this serious problem.

In the 21st century, homeopathy will be utilized to heal a wide assortment of acute and chronic conditions. Chapters 4–13, below, will discuss the applicability of homeopathy to various problems in obstetrics, pediatrics, and women's health and will address such matters as infectious diseases, allergic disorders, chronic conditions, sports medicine, psychological problems, and dental disease. These chapters present a strong case for how and why homeopathic medicines will be the treatment of choice for growing numbers of consumers and health professionals.

Despite the wide applicability of homeopathy, it should be reemphasized that homeopathic medicines complement good medical care. In other words, because most homeopaths are trained medical doctors, and others are usually licensed in some other medical capacity (as, for example, physician assistants, nurses, dentists, naturopaths, chiropractors, and acupuncturists), they generally utilize diagnostic measures similar or identical to those used by conventional doctors to determine what condition a sick person has. They can also refer to appropriate medical specialists, as needed. However, homeopaths have found from clinical experience that their medicines often replace conventional drugs and eliminate the need for heroic medical procedures. Ideally, homeopaths are taking the best of conventional medicine and the best of the natural medicines to create a kind of care that will be commonplace in the 21st century.

One of the most important points about homeopathy is that it will inevitably put the concept of *healing* back into medicine. Doctors and scientists today talk about treating disease, combating illness, suppressing symptoms, and controlling or managing "conditions," often neglecting reference to healing the person. There have recently been more specific references in the conventional medical literature to trying to reestablish homeostasis as a means of restoring health. This subtle but important change in language signifies a deeper change in the approach to healing that increasing numbers of physicians are taking.

In comparison, homeopaths talk about stimulating the body's defenses, catalyzing the immune system, and augmenting the "vital force" when discussing virtually every patient.* As any linguist or therapist will tell you, the words we use are not accidental or without meaning. The fundamental understanding of health, disease, and healing that conventional physicians and homeopaths have is different. Hopefully, as homeopathy develops greater popularity, more conventional physicians will redefine their assumptions about their work.

Besides helping to redefine health and healing by clarifying the difference between suppressing symptoms and curing disease, homeopathy will help us to regain respect for the natural healing powers of the body and teach us ways to augment the body's innate intelligence. It will also provide consumers with a means of taking an active role in their own health and of developing a complementary relationship with their health professionals.

It is no wonder that Gay Gaer Luce, two-time winner of the National Science Writers Award, has proclaimed that "homeopathy is a highly developed health practice that uses a systematic approach to the totality of a person's health. Anyone seeking a fuller understanding of health and healing will find homeopathy extremely important and applicable."[11]

Assumptions About Contemporary and 21st-Century Medicine

One of the best ways to understand one's own culture is to visit another. There are so many things that each of us takes for granted, and because of this we tend to assume that others think, feel, and act in ways similar to our own. Likewise, people commonly assume that the way that conventional physicians think about health, disease, and healing practices is the only appropriate one. This "medical chauvinism" diminishes greatly when one is able to compare it with a different, coherent model of health, disease, and healing. Homeopathic medicine provides this distinctive model.

Because homeopathy provides a coherent model that is distinc-

---

*"Vital force" is the term that 19th-century homeopaths used in reference to the organism's overall interconnected energetic and defense processes, the body's innate wisdom to protect and heal itself.

tive from conventional medicine, it enables people to understand conventional medicine with greater clarity. Although this book is not about conventional medicine, readers hopefully will gain some important insights about modern medicine, too. With this new, larger view of health, disease, and healing, the "medical chauvinism" that presently pervades Western culture will inevitably diminish and fade away.

There are several assumptions about contemporary and 21st-century medicine that underlie much of this book:

1. Despite the various advances in medicine, there is so much more that is not known.
2. Medical care needs to be considerably more scientific than it is at present. Not only must medicine better understand the details of various physiological and psychological processes and how they interact, but it must also comprehend more fully the nature of disease and health. In achieving this goal, doctors should make use of all that is known from other cultures and from different schools of thought within medicine.
3. Conventional physicians are compassionate and even heroic in their efforts to allay pain and suffering, but only in certain circumstances do present-day medical treatments actually cure disease. Although there certainly are exceptions, contemporary medical treatment usually relieves symptoms temporarily but does not necessarily deal with the underlying processes from which the symptoms arise.
4. Side effects from drugs are not really "side" effects but are an integral and often predictable direct effect of the drug upon the human organism. People usually assume that the beneficial effects from a drug are its actions, and that its negative effects are what is called its "side" effects. Actually, drugs simply have effects, and we arbitrarily distinguish those we prefer from those we don't.
5. What was called conventional medicine just thirty years ago would be considered primitive care today, and medical care a hundred years ago would be considered barbaric today. Similarly, what we call conventional medicine today will be considered relatively primitive in the near future and will

probably be considered barbaric in the more distant future. Once this perspective about the continuing evolution of medicine is consciously acknowledged, physicians and scientists will probably not be so dogmatic in their exclusion of unconventional therapies that don't seem to fit within present-day theories of health and disease.[12]

6. 21st-century medicine will focus on methods that stimulate immune and defense responses, rather than on treatments that are primarily symptomatic.

7. Control and suppression of symptoms by pharmocological means will be utilized in the 21st century, but generally not as the treatment of first choice.

8. Treating symptoms with conventional drugs or surgery will be considered "radical therapy," while safer means that aid the body in its own healing will be considered "conservative treatment."

9. Homeopathic medicine will be the primary pharmacological means to stimulate immune and defense responses.

10. "Alternative" medicine will no longer be considered "alternative," but will be an integral part of a comprehensive health care system.

11. Ultimately, a collaborative model of medicine will exist in which physicians and healers of various disciplines collaborate together and in which patients take a more active role as an integral part of the health care team.

Alan Kay, the founder of the Atari Corporation, once said, "The best way to predict the future is to invent it." Perhaps the best way to predict the future of medicine is to practice it. Since homeopathy will be an integral part of this future, utilizing homeopathic medicines is one important step in bringing the future closer to the present.

Notes

1. U.S. Bureau of Census, "Projections of the Population of the United States, by Age, Sex, and Race: 1983–2080," Series P-25, 952 (Washington, D.C.: U.S. Government Printing Office, 1984), p. 7, Table E.

2. *Medical Abstracts Newsletter*, 6 (September 1986): 1.

3. Ibid.

4. Clement Bezold, Rick Carlson, and Jonathan Peck, *The Future of Work and Health* (Dover, Mass.: Auburn House, 1986). (Winner of one of the Book of the Year Awards from *American Health*.)

5. See *Advances: Journal of the Institute for the Advancement of Health*, 16 E. 53rd St., New York, N.Y. 10022. This is the major journal in the field of psychoneuroimmunology.

6. Harris L. Coulter, *Divided Legacy* (Berkeley: North Atlantic Books, 1975), vol. 3, p. 460, n. 147.

7. See Helen Mathews Smith, "The Rebirth of Homeopathy," *MD Magazine*, April 1985, pp. 114–121; *World Homeopathic Directory 1982* (New Delhi: World Homeopathic Links, 1982).

8. René Dubos, *The Mirage of Health* (San Francisco: Harper and Row, 1959), p. 161.

9. See Coulter, *Divided Legacy*, vol. 3; Thomas L. Bradford, *The Logic of Figures or Comparative Results of Homoeopathic and Other Treatments* (Philadelphia: Boericke and Tafel, 1900).

10. K. Steele et al., "Iatrogenic Illness on a General Medical Service at a University Hospital," *New England Journal of Medicine*, 304 (1981): 638–642.

11. Written communication to the author.

12. Michael Baum, a British professor of surgery, has made a similar statement: "What is non-science today may indeed become the science of tomorrow, and with these thoughts in mind the complacencies of both schools of thought must be shaken." ("Science vs. Non-Science in Medicine: Fact or Fiction," *Journal of the Royal Society of Medicine*, 80 [June 1987]: 336–337.)

I

The Science and Art of Homeopathic Medicine

1

A Modern Understanding
of Homeopathic Medicine

Great Britain's Royal Family, Mahatma Gandhi, Mother Teresa, John D. Rockefeller, Sr., Tina Turner, and Yehudi Menuhin don't have much in common, except for the fact that they all have been strong supporters of homeopathic medicine.[1] There is one simple reason that these and other respected individuals the world over have supported homeopathic medicine: it works.

The science and art of homeopathy embody what many people envision as a 21st-century medicine. Homeopathy is a medical approach that respects the wisdom of the body. It is an approach that utilizes medicines that stimulate the body's own immune and defense systems to initiate the healing process. It is an approach that individualizes medicines according to the totality of the person's physical, emotional, and mental symptoms. It is an approach that is widely recognized to be safe. And it is an approach that can be potentially very effective in treating the new types of diseases that are afflicting us now and will affect us in the 21st century.

To understand this science and art, it is first necessary to define some important assumptions that homeopathy has about healing.

Symptoms as Defenses

Too often, physicians and patients alike assume that a person's symptoms *are* the disease and that simply treating these symptoms is the best way to cure the patient. Such treatment is on a par with trying to unplug a car's emergency oil light because it is flashing. Although unplugging the bulb is effective in stopping that irritating flashing light, it does nothing to change the reason it is giving its warning.

The word *symptom* comes from a Greek root and refers to "something that falls together with something else." Symptoms, then, are a sign or signal of something else, and treating them does not necessarily change that "something else."

In 1942, Walter B. Cannon, a medical doctor, wrote *The Wisdom of the Body*.[2] This book, which is a classic in medicine, details the impressive and sophisticated efforts that the body deploys to defend and heal itself. A growing number of physiologists, including Dr. Hans Selye, who is considered to be the father of stress theory, have taken Cannon's work further, recognizing that symptoms are actually efforts of the organism to deal with stress or infection. Rather than viewing symptoms simply as signs of the body's breakdown, these medical doctors see symptoms as defenses of the body that attempt to protect and heal it.[3]

Concepts in new physics offer further support for the notion that living and nonliving systems have inherent self-regulating, self-organizing, and self-healing capacities. This ongoing effort to maintain homeostasis (balance) and to develop higher and higher levels of order and stability has been described in detail by Nobel Prize–winning physicist Ilya Prigogine in *Order Out of Chaos*, by Fritjof Capra in *The Turning Point*, and by Erich Jantsch in *The Self-Organizing Universe*.[4]

Recent research has shown that fevers represent an effort of the organism to try to heal itself. Fever usually accompanies bacterial or viral infection. Physiologist Matthew Kluger and his associates at the University of Michigan Medical School have shown that the body prepares itself to resist infection by creating a fever;

it is then more able to produce interferon (an antiviral substance). Fever also increases white blood cell mobility and activity, instrumental factors in fighting infection.[5]

If fevers are now becoming recognized as adaptive defenses of the body, it is understandable why suppressing them with aspirin is gradually being discouraged.* Using this drug on children with flu or chicken pox is particularly counterproductive, since it also puts them at risk of contracting Reyes Syndrome (a potentially fatal neurological condition).

Modern medical science is recognizing more and more symptoms as adaptive responses of the body. For instance, standard pathology texts define the process of inflammation as the manner in which the body seeks to wall off, heat up, and burn out infective agents or foreign matter.[6] The cough has long been known as a protective mechanism for clearing breathing passages. Diarrhea has been shown to be a defensive effort of the body to remove pathogens or irritants more quickly from the colon.[7] Discharges are understood as the body's way of ridding itself of mucus, dead bacteria, viruses, and cells.

The implications of recognizing that symptoms are efforts of the body to defend itself are significant. Many conventional drugs are specifically prescribed to control or suppress symptoms. As the result of this action, these drugs may well *inhibit* the body's defense and immune processes. Such drugs should be avoided, except in special circumstances.

Homeopathy's Basic Principle: The Law of Similars

It is common knowledge that every plant, mineral, and chemical can cause in overdose its own unique set of physical, emotional,

---

*There are, of course, times when a fever gets so high that it can cause serious, long-term damage to a person's health. A great number of homeopathy's practitioners are trained physicians, and they recognize the importance of heroic medical treatment in select cases. Homeopaths, however, tend to be conservative in treatment and rely on suppressive drugs only when it is medically necessary or when a patient's suffering is extreme.

and mental symptoms. It also is readily acknowledged that individuals, when ill, have their own idiosyncratic physical, emotional, and mental symptom patterns, even when they have the same disease. Homeopathic medicine is a natural pharmaceutical science in which a practitioner seeks to find a substance that would cause in overdose similar symptoms to those a sick person is experiencing. When the match is made, that substance then is given in very small, safe doses, often with dramatic effects.

Homeopaths define the underlying principle for this matching process as the "law of similars." The "law" is not unknown to conventional medicine. Immunizations are based on the principle of similars. No less a person than Dr. Emil Adolph von Behring, the "father of immunology," directly pointed to the origins of immunizations when he asserted: "By what technical term could we more appropriately speak of this influence than by Hahnemann's word 'homeopathy'?"[8] Modern allergy treatment likewise utilizes the homeopathic approach by the use of small doses of allergens in order to create an antibody response.

Conventional medicine also uses homeopathic-like therapy in choosing radiation to treat people with cancer (radiation causes cancer), digitalis for heart conditions (digitalis creates heart conditions), and ritalin for hyperactive children (ritalin is an amphetamine-like drug that normally causes hyperactivity). Other examples are the use of nitroglycerine for heart conditions, gold salts for arthritic conditions, and colchicine for gout.*

It should be remembered that although these conventional medical treatments utilize the homeopathic law of similars, they do not follow other fundamental principles of homeopathy. For example, they are not individually prescribed to the degree of selec-

---

*Few people know that nitroglycerine was first introduced as a medicine by Constantine Hering, a homeopathic physician. For a more detailed history of the use of nitroglycerine in medicine, see W. B. Fye, "Nitroglycerine: A Homeopathic Remedy," *Circulation*, 73 (January 1986): 21–29. Also, for an historical discussion of various homeopathic drugs that have been incorporated into conventional medicine, see Harris Coulter, *Homoeopathic Influences in Nineteenth Century Allopathic Therapeutics* (St. Louis: Formur, 1973).

tivity common in homeopathy, and they are not prescribed in a similar safe, extremely small dose.

The law of similars is also a basic principle of physics, one that many of us may have learned in elementary school. My first-grade teacher showed us magnets and how opposite poles attract while similar poles repel. She also showed us how to recharge a weakened magnet: place similar poles next to each other; eventually the magnet will be recharged and will again repel itself from the other. As in homeopathy, like recharges/regenerates/heals like.

Besides being used in conventional medicine and science, the law of similars has a global and historical basis in healing.[9] In the 4th century B.C., Hippocrates was known to have said: "Through the like, disease is produced, and through the application of the like it is cured."[10] The Delphic Oracle proclaimed the value of the law of similars, stating: "That which makes sick shall heal." Another story from Greek mythology that gives an example of the similars principle in action, though in a magical rather than medicinal way, is the tale of Telephus, a Trojan hero who is speared and then needs to obtain the original spear for his healing.

Paracelsus, a well-known 15th-century physician and alchemist, used the law of similars extensively in his practice and referred to it in his writings. His formulation of the "Doctrine of Signatures" spoke directly of the value in using similars in healing. He affirmed: "You there bring together the same anatomy of the herbs and the same anatomy of the illness into one order. This simile gives you understanding of the way in which you shall heal."[11]

Even Shakespeare recognized the value of similars when he wrote in *Romeo and Juliet:*

> *Tut, man, one fire burns out another's burning;*
> *One pain is lessened by another's anguish,*
> *Turn giddy and be holp by backward turning;*
> *One desperate grief cures with another's languish.*
> *Take thou some new infection to the eye,*
> *And the rank poison of the old will die.*

And Johann Wolfgang Goethe affirmed the special value of similars in his most famous play, *Faust:*

To like things like, whatever one may ail;
there's certain help.

The use of the similars concept has Eastern roots as well. The martial art, aikido, is based on the principle that by using the force of the attacker against himself, a person is better able to defend himself than if he attempts to butt up directly against the attacker's blows. Aikido practitioners are known to blend and flow with the force of the attacker and, without much effort, are able to throw an attacker to the ground. In a similar vein, homeopathic medicines are chosen for their ability to match and mimic the symptoms of the sick person and thereby go *with*, rather than *against*, the body's effort to heal itself. It is thus understandable that Stewart Brand, editor of the *Whole Earth Catalog*, refers to homeopathy as "medical aikido."[12]

The law of similars may indeed have various applications, but its use in healing constitutes the very basis of homeopathic medicine. And its use in healing makes clear and obvious sense; since symptoms are defenses of the body, it is logical to aid rather than suppress them.

The law of similars is not simply a philosophical construct but is a practical guide to prescribing a medicine that will heal. For example, Andrea, a 14-year-old girl, woke up one morning with a sore throat. She said that she felt a lot of swelling and that there was a burning and stinging pain in her throat. Upon further questioning, it was discovered that warm food or drink aggravated the pain, whereas cold food or drink was soothing. Although she was drinking a bit, she was not at all thirsty. She was tearful and even whiny. If one had access to any of the common homeopathic books, one would readily match her symptoms to that of bee venom *Apis mellifica)*. As is widely known, bee venom causes swelling with burning, stinging pain. Further investigation of the toxicological properties of bee venom reveals all of Andrea's other symptoms.

Andrea was given a very small, homeopathically prepared dose of bee venom, and within hours she was feeling completely healthy. Prepared in this way, the homeopathic drug stimulates the appropriate defense response required for the healing.

The beauty of the law of similars is that it not only heals but encourages a respect for the body's wisdom. It teaches us to avoid therapies that suppress symptoms and to seek treatments that truly cure. And it reminds us that there are medicinals that can stimulate the immune and defense systems. The law of similars is one of nature's laws that, when used well, can be one of our highest technologies.

The Importance of Individualization

It is remarkable that people commonly assume that their headache, stomachache, or depression is just like everyone else's. They then assume that they need to take the same drug as others to achieve a cure.

When one talks in depth with several people who have head-aches, it becomes apparent that there are obvious differences between their ailments. One person hurts in the front part of the head, another hurts in the back part. One person has it worse on the left, another on the right. One person says it worsens when moving, another says when lying down. One person likes putting a heating pad on his head, another prefers an ice pack.

Upon further questioning, one discovers that some people with headaches have accompanying digestive problems, while others have dizziness, others have a sore throat, and still others have a backache.

The way homeopaths learn what a homeopathic medicine will cure is through the use of experiments called "drug provings." In these homeopathic drug trials, researchers administer continual doses of a substance to a healthy individual until a reaction to the substance is achieved.* The subject is asked to keep detailed records

---

*Only healthy individuals are used in these experiments. Symptoms experienced by ill people would not be as trustworthy, since it would be uncertain if the symptoms were the result of the substance or a part of the disease process. Provings are usually conducted with the potentized dose of a substance, though the crude dose is also tested. (See my discussion below on "potentization.") Not all people react to the repeated ingestion of microdoses of every substance. Certain people seem to be particularly sensitive to individual medicines.

of symptoms; additional symptoms are discovered through an interview. The subject is instructed to stop ingesting the substance as soon as any particularly discomforting symptom manifests.

Once it is known what symptoms a substance causes, it is then known what it will influence and cure when given in extremely small, specially prepared doses. The information obtained from these drug trials is compiled into *materia medicas* (encyclopedias of drug effects) and *repertories* (books that list symptoms and the substances that have been found to cause and/or cure them).

For technology-minded people, it is obvious that homeopathy is a perfect system for computerization; and, in fact, there are several good computer programs now available for the practicing homeopath. (See Homeopathic Resources in Part III, below.) The various programs are different, but basically one lists the patient's symptoms, and the computer seeks and finds medicines that can cause (and cure) the majority of these symptoms. Although this may sound relatively easy, it should be noted that finding the correct medicine involves more art and judgment than simply looking for a medicine that covers the most symptoms. Ultimately, one searches for the medicine that matches the overall picture, not just the parts, of the person. The computer, then, is not a panacea to homeopathic prescribing, but it is a very useful tool. Although, at present, there are no programs for the general public interested in treating themselves and their families, it is probable that such programs will soon become available.

It is inevitable that some people who become interested in homeopathy will seek to find the homeopathic medicine for specific diseases. They will want to know what medicine is good for headaches, arthritis, premenstrual conditions, insomnia, or a host of other conditions. Homeopathy is actually too scientific for one to assume that there is a single medicine appropriate for everyone. In homeopathy it is essential that the medicine be individually prescribed for the sick person.

There are, of course, some medicines that are more commonly given for certain conditions than others. And some homeopathic medicines are given so often for certain conditions that some people come to view them as "for" that problem. However, it is always possible that a sick individual does not have the symptoms that fit a commonly given medicine, and because of this another medicine is required. It is therefore helpful to take a person's case history in great detail in order to be able to give not just an approximate medicine but an individually chosen one.

Anyone who has gone to a homeopathic practitioner knows that the homeopath asks many questions about the person's chief complaint, minor complaints, and various other physical and psychological symptoms. Homeopaths take pride in their serious interest in and use of the idiosyncratic characteristics of each person. The questions that homeopaths commonly ask include: Is there a time of the day that you feel best or worst or that any specific symptom occurs? How does weather affect you? How do you feel at the seashore or in the mountains? Are there any foods that you crave or to which you feel averse?

Skeptics tend to describe the homeopath's interest in the unique symptoms of the person as evidence that this system is quirky and illogical. And yet, once again, it is now readily accepted in modern science that virtually every organ and enzyme of the body has its own daily rhythm and time of day when it becomes particularly active or inactive. It is now known that geothermal changes can affect brain chemistry and affect physical and psychological states. It is now understood that there are increased negative ions at seashores and mountains that can affect states of health. And it is now recognized that food cravings or aversions may signal certain metabolic states.

Obviously, homeopathy is not a quirky system. It is a highly sophisticated method of individualizing small doses of medicines for a specific person. And the more we begin to understand its principles and methodology, the more we will begin to understand the various subtleties of the human body that presently elude our comprehension.

The Use of Small Doses

Homeopathy's law of similars and its reliance on individual treatment can be readily understood and accepted by most people. Homeopathy's special pharmaceutical process is, however, its most controversial aspect. This process, called "potentization," refers to a specific procedure of serial dilution wherein one part by volume of a medicinal substance is diluted with 99 parts of distilled water or ethyl alcohol, which then is vigorously shaken. One part of this solution is diluted further with 99 parts of distilled water or ethyl alcohol and then shaken again. This process of dilution with shaking may be continued to different strengths, most commonly 3, 6, 9, 12, 30, 200, 1,000, 10,000, 50,000 or 100,000.*

It is initially startling to learn that medicines that have been diluted so many times have any effect. It is even more surprising to learn that homeopaths for the past 200 years have observed that the more a medicine has been potentized—that is, diluted in this fashion—the longer it generally acts, the deeper it usually heals, and the fewer doses tend to be needed.

Although the logic of this may be befuddling at first, there is an impressive amount of clinical experience that verifies it (see "The Present Status of Homeopathy" in Chapter 2, below), research that substantiates it (see Chapter 3, below), and even understandable, nonmystical theories that explain why the small doses work.

Before describing any of the theories for how and why the small doses work, it should be noted that such explanations or theories tend to be of secondary importance to most people who prescribe and take homeopathic medicines. Most people use the medicines because they work—certainly a good enough reason. Also, it should be acknowledged that pharmacologists today do not understand how and why most conventional drugs work, despite all the money spent on research. And finally, theories are not the proving ground for facts. By disproving a theory about why small doses are effective, one does not necessarily disprove homeopathy, only that theory.

In explaining how small doses act, an analogy to music is helpful. It is commonly known that when one plays a "C" note

---

*When a homeopathic medicine is labeled *c*, this means that the medicine was diluted 1:99. When a medicine is labeled *x* or *D*, it was diluted 1:9. When a medicine is described as a *30x*, this means it was diluted 1:9 and vigorously shaken; then diluted again 1:9 and shaken; and this procedure was repeated 30 times. When a medicine is labeled *LM*, it was diluted approximately 1:50,000.

on a piano, other "C" notes reverberate. Even on another piano at the other end of a room, "C" notes still have a hypersensitivity to the "C" resonance. In music theory (and physics), there is a basic principle that two things resonate if, and only if, they are "similar."

In homeopathy a medicine is chosen for its "similarity" to the totality of the person's symptoms. When this similarity exists, a person has a hypersensitivity to the substance. Thus, the small doses may work by some biological version of resonance. Now, the skeptic might assert that when the medicines are potentized beyond a certain point, there probably is not even one molecule remaining.* Homeopaths agree that solutions diluted beyond 24x or 12c may not have any molecules of the original solution, but they assert that "something" remains: the essence of the substance, its resonance, its energy, its pattern.

The concept of pattern is important in biology. In our bodies, 2.5 million red cells die every second, and a similar number are born. After seven years, every cell in one's entire body has been replaced. Although we have new cells, we are still the same person. We are the same because the underlying pattern of our being remains.

Science writer K. C. Cole takes this notion a step further: "Even the ultimate pattern that charts the course of all other patterns in a living being—the double helix of DNA—is only, after all, a collection of atoms and molecules. They too can be (and are) continually replaced. Only the pattern remains."[13]

Although homeopathic medicines may be so dilute as not to have any molecules, a pattern of the substance remains.

José Delgado, a neuroscientist who has studied brain function and behavior, describes the human mind as being like a radio receiver that can receive even very small amounts of stimulation. He notes that reception is possible only if the frequency, amplitude, and other characteristics of electromagnetic signals fall within cer-

---

*Scientists make reference to Avogadro's Law, which basically asserts that in all probability there should not be any molecules remaining after a substance is diluted beyond 6.02 times 10^{-23}. The exact level of ultra-molecularity depends on the concentration of the original substance.

tain ranges.[14]

The sensitivity of an organism to small doses of certain substances is evident throughout nature. Science has recently discovered the existence of pheromones, substances secreted like an odor outside of the body by an individual and perceived by a second individual of the same species. Members of other species do not seem to sense these pheromones. The law of similars in action again.

The homeopathic law of similars is fundamentally a method by which one can find an individually chosen substance to which an organism is most sensitive. When the organism receives this message, its immune and defense systems are catalyzed to begin a curative process. Basic research in immunology, allergy, and physics provides evidence of the regenerative effects of "similars" upon the defense system, but homeopathy has already transformed this pharmacological principle into a sophisticated medical science and art.

James Tyler Kent, a 19th-century American homeopathic physician, made frequent reference to "the innate intelligence of the human organism."[15] In so doing, Kent acknowledged the aspect of the organism that enables it to react curatively to microdoses of correctly chosen substances.

Contemporary homeopath George Vithoulkas explains microdose cures by defining the human body as a magnificent cybernetic system.[16] Such a system has the inherent capacity to always respond to changes with the most effective and efficient response, based on its present abilities. Perhaps astronomer Johannes Kepler described this phenomenon as well as it could be described, centuries before computers, when he said: "Nature uses as little as possible of anything."

R. R. Sharma, a professor of biophysics in India, theorizes that the small doses used in homeopathy are able to cross the blood-brain barrier and cellular and nuclear membranes. Dr. Sharma hypothesizes that more potentized homeopathic medicines may act longer and more deeply than less potentized medicines because they can penetrate these physiological barriers and thereby deliver their therapeutic effects more profoundly.[17]

These modern perspectives on the action of the microdoses have some similarities to the traditional explanation in homeopathy for the action of the medicines. Homeopaths conceptualize a "life force" or "vital force," which they describe as the inherent, under-lying, interconnective, self-healing process of the organism. This bioenergetic force is similar to what the Chinese call "chi," the Japanese call "ki," yogis call "prana," Russian scientists call "bio-plasm," and Star Wars characters call "The Force." Homeopaths theorize that this bioenergetic process is sensitive to the submolec-ular homeopathic medicines. The resonance of the microdose is thought to affect the resonance of the person's life force.

New evidence for how small doses can actually have increased strength was recently reported in *Science News*.[18] A study engaged in by chemists who work for the U.S. Government's National Bureau of Standards and who knew nothing about homeopathy noted that when they shook the coupled molecules of nitric oxide, the units did not weaken and break into parts, but rather devel-oped stronger molecular bonds. One can theorize from this research that the homeopathic process of dilution and succussion (shaking) may actually create superstrong molecules, perhaps superstrong medicines.

Scientists in nonmedical fields are finding value in small-dose applications. For instance, during the oil crisis, Dr. Stanley Ries and his colleagues at Michigan State University used microdoses of a fertilizer to stimulate crop production.[19] As an alternative to petroleum-based fertilizer, Ries used doses of an alcohol derived from alfalfa equivalent to 9x, or, as one journalist reported, a dose of about one jigger of vermouth to 800,000 gallons of gin![20]

Publishing his study in the prestigious *Science* magazine, Ries reported that treated tomatoes yielded 30 percent more fruit than untreated tomatoes, carrots were 21 percent bigger and fatter, asparagus plants were 35–60 percent heavier, sweet corn yields increased by nearly 25 percent, and rice increased in its growth as well as in protein content.

The intelligent use of microdoses is just beginning to be con-sidered. When such research develops to the next stage, new, safer, nontoxic technologies will become available, and we will have a new understanding of natural law.

Understanding the Healing Process

As has been earlier noted, the human body is a remarkable organism that will go to great extremes to protect itself and survive. Our various symptoms are evidence of this process, and our differing symptoms represent different levels of defense that our body is synchronously deploying in an effort to survive.

From their basic assumption that the human being lives on three levels of experience—the physical, emotional, and mental—homeopaths have observed a predictable hierarchy by which any cure of chronic illness takes place. Certain symptoms in each category, depending on their intensities, represent more serious stresses to the defense system than others.

The hierarchy is relatively obvious and may be described here in an oversimplified form. On the physical level, a skin rash, for example, may not be as serious as hepatitis, and hepatitis may not be as serious as heart disease. On the emotional level, a minor irritability is more superficial than a strong anger, and an intense fear of death represents a deeper, more seriously ill condition than either. On the mental level, a slightly poor memory is relatively minor compared to a general state of mental confusion, which itself is less significant than a full-blown schizophrenic state.*

Generally, mental symptoms are regarded as the deepest core of an individual's health, emotional problems are of secondary importance, and physical symptoms of tertiary value. The actual depth of an individual symptom in terms of a person's health is determined by its severity, frequency, and degree of impact on limiting the person's freedom to be and act at his or her potential. Thus, any serious or persistent physical symptoms can be considered deeper diseases than emotional or mental symptoms if they threaten basic survival or make living very difficult.

Constantine Hering, M.D. (1800–1880), the father of Ameri-

---

*Symptoms on the mental level might be defined as disturbances in a person's cognitive functioning, sense of self, sense of connectedness with the world, or willpower.

can homeopathy, was one of the first observers to make note of specific ways that healing progresses. He made three observations of the healing process, which he asserted should be understood together as a unitary pattern, and homeopaths have dubbed his observations "Hering's Law of Cure." First, he observed that the human body seeks to externalize disease—to dislodge it from more serious, internal levels to more superficial, external levels. Someone with asthma may develop an external skin rash as part of the curative process. Or someone with a headache may undergo a day or two of fever and sweating as a part of his cure. A person with emotional or mental symptoms may experience different and less serious emotional or mental problems or physical symptoms during his curative process. Sadly, most conventional medical doctors treat each symptom as a unique and unconnected phenomenon. A person's skin rash generally will be treated with cortisone, thus suppressing it—and possibly reactivating the person's asthma. The mentally ill person's new physical symptom is also suppressed, leading to a recurrence of the mental illness.

Hering's second observation was that healing progresses from the top of the body to the bottom. Thus, a person with arthritis in many joints will generally notice relief in the upper part of the body before the lower part. An understanding of this aspect of healing helps homeopaths to differentiate true cures from temporary relief or placebo responses.

Hering's third observation was that healing proceeds in the reverse order of the appearance of the symptoms. Thus, the most recent symptoms will generally be the first to be healed. For this reason, in the process of cure a person may sometimes reexperience symptoms that he or she previously suffered from (generally those symptoms that were suppressed or never really healed). Needless to say, homeopaths are pleased when a person informs them that one of their old symptoms has returned. Although these old symptoms may be irritating, homeopaths will avoid suppressing them. They are usually only experienced for a short period of time, and when they depart this time the person usually experiences a significantly higher level of health.

These three observations of the healing process are not meant to be thought of as universal laws, but as general guiding principles that help us to understand if a patient's health is improving or deteriorating.

Homeopaths are not the only ones to have recognized these laws of cure. Acupuncturists have witnessed aspects of them for thousands of years. Naturopaths and psychotherapists commonly have noted that their patients reexperience old physical or psychological symptoms in the process of healing.

Hering's Law of Cure represents a significant development in medicine. Most conventional physicians and even many "alternative" practitioners evaluate a person's state of health by the person's main symptom. If this symptom goes away, they generally assume that their therapy "worked," even though some new symptom must now be treated. Most practitioners are not working from a model of health that defines the curative process. Hering's Law of Cure is a unique, holistic assessment tool that can be used to evaluate the progress of the healing process over time.

Homeopathic Typologies: The Bodymind Personalities

Clinical psychologists acknowledge the existence of varying personality types; likewise, physical therapists and sports trainers who study the body find variations of body types. Homeopaths assert that body and mind are inseparable, and they posit the necessity of looking at "bodymind" types. A homeopathic medicine is generally given not simply for a symptom or a disease but for an entire pattern or constellation of physical and psychological symptoms.

Homeopaths acknowledge certain groupings of bodymind symptom patterns that a person has and that correspond with the sensitivity of a particular homeopathic medicine. The word *symptom* is here most broadly defined as any sensation that is discomforting or that limits a person's physical or psychological functions. Homeopaths also inquire into what factors (or "modalities") seem to aggravate or ameliorate these sensations. In addition to prescribing on the basis of these factors, a homeopath may utilize information about the person's body type, temperament, disposition, and behavioral tendencies to determine the appropriate medicine.

Dr. Francisco Eizayaga, an Argentinian urologist and internationally respected homeopath, has helped to differentiate the various symptoms and characteristics of a person to find the correct medicine. Dr. Eizayaga has asserted that a "constitutional medicine" is prescribed primarily according to a person's genetic endowment and deep-seated psychological tendencies. A "fundamental medicine" is prescribed according to the functional symptoms that represent the organism's response to the various stresses it is experiencing.* Dr. Eizayaga notes that fundamental states may change and pile up on each other like concentric skins of an onion. Dr. Eizayaga also differentiates the treatment of organic pathology from constitutional or fundamental states, though such a discussion is beyond the scope of an introductory book.[21]

Homeopaths identify certain patterns of symptoms with the medicines that have cured them. There is, for instance, the "Phosphorus type," the "Sulphur type," the "Arsenicum (arsenic) type," and the "Natrum mur (salt) type." Each of these typologies refers not only to a type of headache, for instance, but also to those factors that make that headache better or worse, other physical symptoms that may be related to it, past or present symptoms and diseases, food cravings or aversions, sensitivity to temperature and weather, energy levels at varying times of the day, sweating tendencies, stool and urination characteristics, menstrual patterns, emotional and mental states, and behavioral propensities.

After a homeopath completes a thorough interview, he or she seeks to find a medicine that matches the "essence" of the person's totality of symptoms. The word *essence* is important here, since homeopathy is the science of finding the medicine that is most "similar" to the person. It is not necessary to match every symptom the person has with those symptoms that the substance causes. Rather, it is enough to find a substance that matches the

---

*Many homeopaths do not make a distinction between constitutional and fundamental medicines. They generally refer to the "constitutional medicine" as the one that fits a long-standing set of symptoms that a person experiences, and to the "acute medicine" as that which fits transitory disease states. For ease of discussion in forthcoming chapters, reference will be made only to the "constitutional medicine" when discussing the treatment of the chronically ill based on their totality of symptoms.

essence of the person's characteristics.

Once one's constitutional or fundamental medicine is selected and administered, not only is the person's chief complaint greatly reduced, but he or she generally feels better in many ways, physically and psychologically. Although a person may actually be cured after a single dose of the correct constitutional or fundamental medicine, more often the medicine may start the curative process, and a series of medicines will be required to complete it. As the person heals and changes, a new fundamental picture often emerges, bringing with it the requirement of a new medicine. Some homeopaths believe that one's constitutional medicine never changes, whereas others feel that it can.

Some laypersons find great pleasure in looking for their own, their family's, and their friends' constitutional medicines. The most popular and useful books for this endeavor are Catherine Coulter's *Portraits of Homoeopathic Medicines*, Edward C. Whitmont's *Psyche and Substance: Essays on Homeopathy in the Light of Jungian Psychology*, James Tyler Kent's *Lectures on Homoeopathic Materia Medica*, D.M. Gibson's *Studies of Homoeopathic Remedies*, and Margaret Tyler's *Drug Pictures*. (See "Sources of Homeopathic Books, Tapes, and General Information" in Part III, below.)

The search for a constitutional medicine requires one's intellectual and intuitive capacities; one must be part detective, part psychologist, and part investigative reporter. Despite the challenge of this process, it is not recommended that one prescribe a constitutional or fundamental medicine for oneself, for several reasons. First, it is the consensus in the homeopathic community that laypersons can learn to treat themselves for nonemergency acute conditions, but that the complexity of treating chronic conditions and of providing follow-up treatment requires professional supervision. Since the treatment of chronic conditions usually involves a sequence of prescriptions (either repetition of the same medicine at the same or a different potency or another medicine entirely), only those with deeper knowledge of homeopathic principles and materia medica should engage in it.

Another reason that laypersons should not prescribe constitutional or fundamental medicines is that such medicines can sometimes create a healing crisis during which certain symptoms get worse. If the layperson does not know how to deal with this situation, the person receiving treatment will not get the best benefit from the homeopathic medicine.

Although it is not recommended for laypersons to prescribe medicines for their own or others' chronic states, it may still be worthwhile for them to study the different homeopathic types and to give their opinion to the practitioner as to what medicine might be considered. Even so, there are three caveats. The first is that people who study certain medicines may create for themselves by self-suggestion symptoms specific to a particular medicine. Second, some people may exaggerate certain symptoms in order to fit a medicine. And third, some people like to think of themselves as particular "nice person" medicine types, such as *Sulphur, Phosphorus,* or *Pulsatilla,* and angrily deny that they are the more irritable types, such as *Nux vomica, Sepia,* or *Arsenicum.* The potential for bias here is obvious.

A constitutional homeopathic medicine may significantly reduce certain physical or psychological tendencies so that they limit the person's capacity to do and be his or her best. A homeopathic medicine may reduce the extreme symptoms that stress the bodymind and increase the overall physical and psychological strength within each of us, but it cannot change those propensities and idiosyncratic characteristics that make each of us unique.

Dr. Edward Whitmont sheds light on this phenomenon by describing a humorous pantomime called "The Hair in the Soup," which depicts the reactions of four different people to finding a hair in their soup. The first flies into a rage and throws the soup at the waiter. The second expresses disgust, shrugs it off, and leaves the restaurant whistling a tune. The third begins crying because bad things always happen to him. The fourth looks at the hair, leaves it where it is, goes on eating, and, after finishing, orders another bowl. Dr. Whitmont notes that these four reactions represent four classic temperaments. Each reaction is a reflex behavior that, like a simple cough, is automatic and that each person develops as a defense response. One might submit to various therapies to become more conscious of his or her own behavioral patterns, but the attempt to change one's nature is usually ineffective and tends to generate its own set of symptoms. The angry person who throws his soup at the waiter will, after a homeopathic medicine, still feel angry, though he may direct the fire of this emotion in a more constructive way. If, on the other hand, the person seeks to ignore or suppress the passion he feels, his body and mind will pay another price for it. Thus, homeopathic medicines may eliminate various physical and psychological symptoms, but they cannot alter a person's innate tendencies.

Treating one's overall constitutional state is both ancient and futuristic in concept. It has been a part of medicine at least since the times of Hippocrates, and it has often been a preferred approach to simply treating a specific symptom or disease. Today, constitutional therapies are the ones that aid the immune and defense systems and have special value in preventing and treating various acute and chronic conditions. The homeopathic method of individualizing a medicine based on the totality of the person's symptoms is a sophisticated 21st-century science.

Unconventional Approaches to Homeopathy

This book primarily describes the traditional or classical approach to homeopathy—that is, the use of a single medicine, given in microdose, based on a person's physical and psychological symptoms. However, from homeopathy's beginnings, some homeopaths have used more than a single medicine at a time, and different others have used instruments to determine a person's homeopathic microdose.

The best-known unconventional usage of the homeopathic medicines is "combination medicines," or "complexes." A combination medicine is a mixture of three to eight low-potency (usually 3x to 12x) homeopathic medicines mixed together, each chosen because it is a commonly used medicine for a specific condition. These combination medicines are often sold in health food stores and are named for the specific disease or symptom the medicine is thought to help. For example, there are combination medicines for "teething," "insomnia," "cough," or "hay fever." Sometimes, a manufacturer will describe the medicine by its acton, such as "Calms" for its application in a hyperactive or nervous condition. Combination medicines are only available for non-life-threatening conditions.

Great numbers of people have their first introduction to homeopathy by using combination medicines because of their widespread availability. These experiences are often quite positive. Effective treatment for recurrent symptoms, however, generally requires the use of a single, individually prescribed homeopathic medicine. Such individualized treatment can deal with the problem as well as the underlying condition. Still, the combination medicines are invaluable when the seemingly correct individual medicine isn't readily available or when one does not know which single homeopathic medicine is appropriate.

Another unconventional use of the homeopathic medicines is the application of two or more individual medicines at a time, each of which is taken at different times of the day. "Pluralism," as this practice is called, is commonly used by practitioners in Europe; it is a method by which the homeopath prescribes one medicine for one group of symptoms, a second for another group, and a third for yet another. European homeopaths claim good results with this approach, though no formal research has compared it with the classical approach to homeopathy.

Besides the above-described unconventional use of homeopathic medicines, there are also unconventional ways to find the correct medicine(s). With the development of modern technology, new electronic equipment has been applied to find the appropriate treatment. The practitioner assesses the person's health by placing electrodes on acupuncture points and measuring electrical conductance. On a 100-point scale, which is what is used on most of these instruments, a reading of 50 has been determined to be normal or healthy, while a reading over 50 indicates hyperactivity or inflammation, and a reading under 50 indicates underactivity or degeneration. The practitioner then compares this reading with that done while the patient holds onto bottles containing varying homeopathic medicines. The medicine(s) that is found to normalize the readings is thought to be helpful for the sick individual.

Some physicians in Europe and the United States have used electronic equipment to determine homeopathic medicines for over twenty years. No formal studies have yet been completed to measure the effectiveness of medicines prescribed with the aid of these machines.

A small group of practitioners utilize a pendulum to determine the correct homeopathic medicine. Using a pendulum as a
dowsing instrument, the practitioner finds the correct medicine
for the person.

Dr. Albert Abrams, the Dean of Clinical Medicine at Stan-
ford Medical School in the early 1900s, extended the use of pendulums by developing a machine that measured the subtle emana-
tions of the body and of medicines. Initially referred to as "The
Electronic Reactions of Abrams," this system later became known
as "radionics." Although radionics is derided by critics today as
the epitome of quackery, Sir James Barr, a past President of the
British Medical Assocation who duplicated some of Abrams's experiments, described him as one of the greatest medical geniuses
of the early twentieth century.[22]

More recently, another method to find the correct homeopathic medicine is "applied kinesiology," the testing of muscle
strength to assess the health of organ systems that are thought to
correspond to such muscles. The practitioner tests muscle strength
and compares it to the strength measured when the patient holds
onto a bottled homeopathic medicine. The use of applied kinesiology, like most unconventional diagnostic and therapeutic
methods, has not been adequately tested to determine its accuracy
or efficacy.

Although some practitioners think that these unconventional
methods objectively verify the correct homeopathic medicines,
even the experienced users of these methods acknowledge that
strong subjective factors play an intimate role in assessing and
treating people. Since the various unconventional methods that
help to find the correct homeopathic medicine have uncertain ac-
cracy, it is prudent to complement their use with conventional
homeopathic case-taking and case analysis.

The Limitations and Risks
of Homeopathic Medicine

Homeopathic medicines are indeed powerful tools, but they are
not effective in treating all diseased states. Some conditions do not

respond to microdoses because they require surgical intervention, some require immediate and certain relief of symptoms, others are addressed by simple nutritional or lifestyle changes, still others are relieved only upon reduced exposure to certain environmental stresses—and then there are those persons who don't experience any improvement from homeopathic medicine for unknown reasons.

At the turn of the century, some of America's leading surgeons were homeopathic physicians. Homeopaths are thus not against surgery, since they, like other medical professionals, recognize the special value of surgery in certain circumstances. Homeopathic medicines, however, can be of great value in reducing the need for surgery in certain circumstances, and at other times the medicines can be invaluable in helping persons heal after surgery is completed.

Homeopathic medicines may also not be appropriate for some symptoms that are life-threatening and call for immediate, sometimes heroic, means of treatment. Certain cases of asthma in which breathing is significantly impaired, meningitis that requires immediate antibiotic treatment to avoid possible brain damage or death, and various other conditions require conventional medical treatment to assure survival. This is not to say that homeopathic medicines are of no value in these situations. In fact, homeopathic medicines may reduce the need for conventional medical treatment even in some of these difficult cases. Microdoses may effectively treat a serious attack of asthma, may cure the serious infection without the need for antibiotics, and may rapidly relieve various other life-threatening symptoms. However, since the homeopathic medicines require strict individualization to obtain the best results, one cannot always depend on them for rapid, effective relief of symptoms. There is a consensus among homeopaths that homeopathic medicines can still be used in emergencies, either on the way to the doctor or hospital and/or in conjunction with heroic conventional medical treatments.

Homeopathic medicines are also ineffective in treating some conditions that cry out for simple nutrition and lifestyle changes. A woman may be anemic from a lack of iron in her diet. Homeopathic medicines may be prescribed to deal with some of her symptoms and may even be used to help her assimilate iron from her food more efficiently; but until she gets iron, she may experience persistent symptoms.

Exposure to environmental toxins is becoming a major modern problem. Although homeopathic medicines may be effective in helping a person to reestablish health after exposure to many toxins, real improvement in health is not likely if exposure continues. For instance, a woman with a skin rash went to a homeopathic physician. From her symptoms, the doctor prescribed *Sulphur 30*. The condition temporarily worsened in a classic response according to Hering's Law, then got better, only to return within two weeks. The homeopath gave a stronger dose of *Sulphur*, and the woman once again experienced a similar pattern of exacerbation, relief, and return of her symptoms. Upon obtaining more detail about the woman's job at a food processing plant, the physician discovered that she worked at a dried fruit plant that sprays sulphur on the fruit as a preservative. She was experiencing a sulphur "proving." Her skin finally improved after she changed jobs.

Probably the greatest frustration for a homeopath (and for the patients as well) are those people who, for some uncertain reason, do not respond effectively to homeopathic medicines. Homeopaths often initially assume that the cause of the lack of reaction is that they have not correctly analyzed the case and thus are not giving the correct medicine. Experienced homeopaths know that certain medicines sometimes are valuable when the indicated medicine does not cure. Since it is generally recommended to try these medicines one at a time and allow a month or more between medicines, finding an effective remedy may take several months.* When people with chronic indigestion, headaches, arthritis, or other persistent symptoms are not receiving adequate treatment

---

*Different schools of thought in homeopathy recommend varying lengths of time between different medicines and doses. Some homeopaths prescribe daily doses of a medicine and may change the dose or the medicine at any time, while others prescribe a single dose or a couple of doses and then wait one or more months before changing the dose or the medicine. Generally, those homeopaths who give repeated doses of medicine in a week or a month prescribe low-potency medicines— that is, the 3rd, 6th, 9th, 12th, or 18th potency.

with conventional drugs, delay is not a major problem, since they have already been waiting for curative care for years or even decades. But a patient in pain and discomfort might understandably seek an alternative to homeopathic care before a "similimum" (most similar medicine) can be found.

When careful analysis of a patient's health history, present lifestyle, and potential environmental exposures does not indicate any obvious reason for nonresponse to a microdose, homeopaths may either consult with another homeopath or refer the patient to some other type of health practitioner.

People often ask: Are there conditions that homeopathy treats most effectively, and with which conditions does it not tend to have great success? These are difficult questions that can best be answered by the cliché that homeopathy does not treat diseases, only people. Case histories in homeopathic books and journals describe successful treatment of just about every acute and chronic disease. Many homeopaths assume that there are no incurable diseases, only incurable people.

These parameters are quite simplistic, since a large number of chronic diseases become incurable once they have progressed to a certain stage. Homeopathic medicines may then alleviate pain and discomfort and may stop or slow down the pathological process, but it is questionable if cure is possible under any kind of treatment.

As for the dangers of the homeopathic medicines, it is widely recognized that their greatest danger is only that they may sometimes delay the use of other potentially effective medical treatments. Since most homeopaths are medical doctors or other licensed medical professionals, they generally know when conventional medical care is required or when referral to a specialist is indicated.

Another potential danger of homeopathic medicines arises if a person continues to take a medicine when it is not indicated. A small percentage of such people may experience a "proving"—the symptoms produced in overdose of the substance. These symptoms may occur, as previously described, even with high potencies. Homeopaths do not consider the symptoms of a proving to be a major danger, since they usually end shortly after the person stops taking the medicine. Some homeopaths stop a proving by prescribing the same medicine in a higher (more dilute) potency, and some homeopaths give a medicine that is known to antidote the symptoms of the medicine being proven. Because a proving is possible when a person is not taking the correct medicine, it is recommended not to take a medicine longer than one week unless under professional homeopathic care.

The first time an American medical journal ever published a case suggesting that there is danger in taking homeopathic medicines was in a recent letter to the editor of the *New England Journal of Medicine*.[23] In the case reported, a patient took eight doses in two hours, as recommended by a chiropractor, and shortly thereafter experienced severe epigastric pains, which was later diagnosed as pancreatitis (a potentially dangerous disease). It should be noted, however, that the remedy prescribed by the chiropractor was a "combination medicine" (with nineteen different ingredients) and that it was prescribed for the treatment of cancer. Although the patient's health history was not described in the letter, one might assume that he was not healthy prior to treatment, and one should not necessarily assume that the medicine caused this condition.

There is a consensus that homeopathic medicines are safe, though, like carrot juice, vitamins, and many "natural" substances, they can be misused. Homeopathy is promoted by the National Center of Homeopathy as "The Safer Medicine." There is little disagreement on this fact.

Summary and Conclusion

Homeopathy is a sophisticated medical science that individualizes a substance based on the totality of a person's symptoms. A person's unique pattern of symptoms, his or her headache, stomach ache, constipation, low energy in the morning, sensitivity to cold, irritability at the slightest cause, and fear of heights are all interrelated. No matter what the individual symptoms are, they are recognized as primarily an intrinsic effort of the organism to adapt to and deal with various internal or external stresses. Methods that simply suppress, control, or manage symptoms should be avoided, since such therapies compromise the innate tendency of the organism to defend and heal itself. The side effects that these suppressive treatments cause are actually direct effects of the treatment. Homeopathic medicines, on the other hand, are prescribed to aid the organism in its highly sophisticated efforts to heal itself. Inherent in the homeopathic approach is a basic respect for the body's wisdom; it is thus no wonder that it is a safer medicine.

At a time in our civilization when it is essential to develop practices that strengthen the immune and defense systems, homeopathic medicine is quite naturally gaining popularity. Homeopathy embodies the characteristics of a medical science that one could hope and dream for in the 21st century. And the best news is that we do not have to wait until the 21st century to draw upon its benefits.

Notes

1. The Royal Family has been intimately involved in homeopathic medicine dating back to the 1830s, when Queen Adelaide sought homeopathic care from Dr. Ernst Stapf, a colleague of Dr. Samuel Hahnemann. For further information, see "Homoeopathy: The Royal Key," *Homoeopathy: Journal of the British Homoeopathic Association*, February 1987, pp. 18–21. Mahatma Gandhi was once quoted as saying: "Homeopathy cures a greater number of cases than any other method of treatment." (From a speech on August 30, 1936, quoted in *World Homoeopathic Directory 1982* [New Delhi: World Homoeopathic Links, 1982], p. 32.) John D. Rockefeller, Sr., was known to be under homeopathic care for at least fifteen years of his life. He once described homeopathy as "a progressive and aggressive step in medicine." (A. Nevins, *John D. Rockefeller: The Heroic Age of American Enterprise* [New York: Scribner's, 1940], vol. 2, p. 263.) Tina Turner has been vocal in her support of homeopathy, as mentioned in her autobiography, *I, Tina* (New York: Avon, 1986), and in Maureen Orth's "Tina," *Vogue*, May 1985, pp. 318ff. Yehudi Menuhin's support for homeopathy is epitomized by the fact that he is the President of the Hahnemann Society, one of the major homeopathic organizations in Great Britain.

2. Walter B. Cannon, *The Wisdom of the Body* (New York: Norton, 1942).

3. Hans Selye, *The Stress of Life*, revised edition (New York:

McGraw-Hill, 1978), p. 12.

4. Ilya Prigogine and Isabelle Stengers, *Order Out of Chaos* (New York: Bantam, 1984); Fritjof Capra, *The Turning Point* (New York: Simon and Schuster, 1982); Erich Jantsch, *The Self-Organizing Universe* (Oxford, England: Pergamon, 1980).

5. Matthew Kluger, "Fever," *Pediatrics*, 66 (November 1980): 720–724; idem, "Fever: Effect of Drug-Induced Antipyresis on Survival," *Science*, 193 (July 16, 1976): 237–239; idem, "Fever and Survival," *Science*, 188 (April 11, 1975): 166–168.

6. See William Boyd, *An Introduction to the Study of Disease* (Philadelphia: Lea and Febiger, 1972), pp. 95–110.

7. H. L. DuPont and R. B. Hornick, "The Adverse Effect of Lomotil Therapy in Shigellosis," *JAMA*, 226 (December 24, 1971): 1525–28.

8. Emil Adolph von Behring, *Modern Phthisia-Genetic and Phthisia-Therapeutic Problems in Historical Illumination* (New York, 1906), section 5; originally published in *Beitrage zur Experimentellen Therapie*, 2 (1906). Also see Otto E. Guttentag, "Homeopathy in the Light of Modern Pharmacology," *Clinical Pharmacology and Therapeutics*, 7 (1966): 426.

9. See Linn Boyd, *A Study of the Simile in Medicine* (Philadelphia: Boericke and Tafel, 1936).

10. Quoted in Maesimund Panos and Jane Heimlich, *Homeopathic Medicine at Home* (Los Angeles: J. P. Tarcher, 1980), p. 11. For further references to various places in the Hippocratic writings that discuss the similars principles, see Harris L. Coulter, *Divided Legacy—The Patterns Emerge: Hippocrates to Paracelsus* (Washington, D.C.: Wehawken, 1975), pp. 205–206.

11. Quoted in Coulter, *Divided Legacy*, vol. 3, p. 432. Although the Doctrine of Signatures has some resemblance to the homeopathic law of similars, the signatures principle, which is based on analytical interpretation, is not as precise as the homeopathic method, which utilizes drug trials and "provings" to determine the symptoms that each substance will heal.

12. Steward Brand, *Whole Earth Epilog* (Baltimore: Penguin, 1974), p. 606.

13. K. C. Cole, *Sympathetic Vibrations* (New York: Bantam, 1985), p. 280.

14. Kathleen McAuliffe, "The Mind Fields," *Omni*, January 1985, pp. 42–44.

15. James Tyler Kent, *Lectures on Homoeopathic Philosophy* (Berkeley: North Atlantic Books, 1979).

16. George Vithoulkas, *The Science of Homeopathy* (New York: Grove Press, 1980), p. 87.

17. R. R. Sharma, "Homoeopathy Today: A Scientific Appraisal," *British Homoeopathic Journal*, 75 (October 1986): 231–236.

18. I. Amato, "Molecular Divorce Gives Strange Vibes," *Science News*, November 1, 1986, pp. 277–278.

19. Stanley Ries et al., "Triacontanol: A New Naturally Occurring Plant Growth Regulator," *Science*, 195 (1977): 1339–41.

20. David Perlman, "Chance Discovery of a Magic Fertilizer," *San Francisco Chronicle*, November 15, 1977, p. 1.

21. Francisco X. Eizayaga, *Tratado de Medicina Homeopatica* [Treatise on Homeopathic Medicine] (Buenos Aires: Ediciones Marecel, 1981). A set of tapes in English on Dr. Eizayaga's basic concepts is available from Homeopathic Educational Services, 2124 Kittredge St., Berkeley, CA 94704.

22. Edward W. Russell, *Report on Radionics* (Suffolk, England: Neville Spearman, 1973), p. 17.

23. H. D. Kerr and G. W. Yarborough, "Pancreatitis Following Ingestion of a Homeopathic Preparation," *New England Journal of Medicine*, 314 (June 19, 1986): 642–643.

2

A Condensed History
of Homeopathy

The history of homeopathy combines the high drama and intrigue commonly found in the best efforts of the silver screen. It is a film waiting to happen.

Homeopathy became spectacularly popular in the United States and Europe in the 1800s, and its strongest advocates included European royalty, American entrepreneurs, literary giants, and religious leaders. But at the same time that it was gaining widespread popularity, it became the object of deep-seated animosity and vigilant opposition from establishment medicine. The conflict between homeopathy and orthodox medicine was protracted and bitter. We know who won the first round of this conflict. We await the results of the second round. Hopefully, we will soon discover that a "fight" over healing is inappropriate and that various approaches to healing are all necessary to build a comprehensive and effective health care system.

The history of homeopathy begins with the discoveries of its founder Samuel Hahnemann (1755–1843), a German physician. Hahnemann first coined the word *homeopathy* (*homoios* in Greek means "similar," *pathos* means "suffering") to refer to the pharmacological principle, the law of similars, that is its basis. Actually, the law of similars was previously described by Hippocrates and Paracelsus and was utilized by many cultures, including the Mayans, Chinese, Greeks, Native American Indians, and Asian

Indians,[1] but it was Hahnemann who codified the law into a systematic medical science.

Hahnemann's first comments about the general applicability of the law of similars came in 1789, when he translated a book by William Cullen, one of the leading physicians of the era. At one point in the book, Cullen ascribed the usefulness of Peruvian bark (cinchona) in treating malaria to its bitter and astringent properties. Hahnemann wrote a bold footnote in his translation, disputing Cullen's explanation. Hahnemann asserted that the efficacy of Peruvian bark must derive from some other factor, since he noted that there were other substances and mixtures of substances decidedly more bitter and more astringent than Peruvian bark that were not effective in treating malaria. He then described his own taking of repeated doses of this herb until his body responded to its toxic dose with fever, chills, and other symptoms similar to malaria. Hahnemann concluded that the reason this herb was beneficial was because it caused symptoms similar to those of the disease it was treating.[2]

This account epitomizes Hahnemann. First, he was translating Cullen's work, with suggests that he was one of the more respected translators of his day. By the time he was only 24, Hahnemann could read and write in at least seven languages. He ultimately translated over twenty major medical and scientific texts. This story reveals Hahnemann as both an avid experimenter and a respected chemist. He had authored a four-volume set of books called *The Pharmaceutical Lexicon*, which was considered one of the standard reference texts for apothecaries/pharmacists of his day.[3] And this account also reveals Hahnemann as an audacious rebel. He was unafraid to speak his mind, even if it meant correcting the analysis of a very respected physician. He was unafraid to question commonly accepted truths. And he had enough initiative to seek his own alternative explanations.

After translating Cullen's work, Hahnemann spent the next six years actively experimenting on himself, his family, and a small but growing group of followers. In 1796, he wrote about his experiences with the law of similars in *Hufeland's Journal*, a respected medical journal in Germany.[4] Coincidentally, in 1798, Edward Jenner discovered the value of giving small doses of cowpox to people in an effort to immunize them against smallpox. Whereas Jenner's work was generally accepted into orthodox medicine, Hahnemann's work was not. In fact, there was so much antagonism to Hahnemann and the new school of medical thought he called homeopathy that entire medical journals were called *Anti-Homoeopathic Archives* or *Anti-Organon* (*Organon* was the title of the book that Hahnemann wrote as the primary text on the homeopathic art and science).[5]

Hahnemann was particularly disliked by the apothecaries, because he recommended the use of only one medicine at a time and prescribed only limited doses of it.[6] Because he recommended only small doses of each medicine, the apothecaries could not charge much for them. And because each medicine required careful preparation, Hahnemann found that the apothecaries did not always make them correctly or intentionally gave his patients different medicines. As he grew to distrust the apothecaries, he chose to dispense his own medicines, which was illegal at the time in Germany. The apothecaries then accused Hahnemann of "entrenching upon their privileges by the dispensing of medicines."[7] Arrested in Leipzig in 1820, he was found guilty and forced to move.

He moved to Kothen, where he was delegated special permission to practice and to dispense his own medicines by Grand Duke Ferdinand, one of the many members of European royalty who supported homeopathy.[8]

Despite the persecution, homeopathy continued to grow. It grew not just because it offered a systematic approach to treating sick people but also because orthodox medicine was often ineffective and even dangerous. There is general agreement among medical historians today that orthodox medicine of the 1700s and 1800s frequently caused more harm than good.[9]

Bloodletting and the application of leeches were common practice up to the mid-1800s. One French doctor bloodlet so much that some people jokingly estimated that he spilled more blood in his medical practice than was spilled throughout the entire Napoleonic Wars.[10] Benjamin Rush, considered the father of American medicine, asserted that bloodletting was useful in all general and chronic disease.[11] As many as 41 million leeches were imported into France in 1833 alone.[12] And in the United States, one firm imported 500,000 leeches in 1856; its nearest competitor imported 300,000.[13] Besides bloodletting and leeches, orthodox physicians used medicines made from mercury, lead, arsenic, and various strong herbs to help purge the body of foreign disease-causing matter.

The combination of poor medical care and prejudicial reaction against homeopathy is certainly understandable in light of medical education at the time. Nathan Smith Davis, who was the driving force in the creation of the American Medical Association, described medical education in 1845:

> All the young man has to do is gain admittance in the office of some physician, where he can have access to a series of ordinary medical text-books, and see a patient perhaps once a month, with perhaps a hasty post-mortem examination once a year; and in the course of three years thus spent, one or two courses of lectures in the medical colleges, where the whole science of medicine, including anatomy, physiology, chemistry, materia medica, pathology, practice of medicine, medical jurisprudence, surgery, and midwivery are all crowded upon his mind in the short space of *sixteen* weeks, . . . and his education, both primary and medical, is deemed complete.[14]

Despite the fact that historians and scientists today consider medicine of the 18th and 19th centuries as unscientific and even barbaric, orthodox physicians had the audacity to call homeopathy "quackery," "unscientific," "cultish," and "devilish."

The Opposition to Homeopathy

Homeopathy posed a serious threat to entrenched medicine. Orthodox physicians criticized herbalists, midwives, and various other "nonregular" practitioners because they were not medically trained. Homeopaths, however, could not be discredited as unlearned, since they had been graduated from many of the same medical schools as "regular" physicians. In fact, many of the initial practitioners of homeopathy were graduates from Harvard, Dartmouth, and other prestigious medical schools.[15]

Orthodox medicine was also threatened because homeopathy offered an integrated, coherent, systematic basis for its therapeutic

practice. In his Pulitzer Prize–winning book *The Social Transformation of American Medicine*, Paul Starr noted: "Because homeopathy was simultaneously philosophical and experimental, it
seemed to many people to be more rather than less scientific than
orthodox medicine."[16]

One of the most important reasons that orthodox physicians
and drug companies disliked homeopathy was that inherent in the
homeopathic approach was a sharp critique of the use of conventional drugs. Homeopaths were primarily critical of the suppressive
nature of these drugs. They felt that the drugs simply masked the
person's symptoms, creating deeper, more serious diseases. Homeopaths also noted that this masking of symptoms made it more difficult for them ultimately to find the correct medicine, since the
person's idiosyncratic symptoms are the primary guide to the individual selection of the medicine.

Perhaps the most important reason that conventional physicians disliked homeopathy and homeopaths was well expressed at
a 1903 AMA meeting by one of the more respected orthodox physicians. "We must," he said, "admit that we never fought the homeopath on matters of principles; we fought him because he came
into the community and got the business."[17] Although most physicians, past or present, will not so easily admit this, economic issues
play a major role in what is practiced and what is allowed to be
practiced.

Hahnemann's principles therefore posed a philosophical, clinical, and economic threat to orthodox medicine.

Homeopathy began growing in the New World shortly after
Hans Gram, a Danish homeopath, emigrated to the United States
in 1825. It expanded so rapidly that the homeopaths decided to
create a national medical society. In 1844, they organized the
American Institute of Homeopathy, which became America's first
national medical society.[18] Partially in response to the growth of
the homeopaths, in 1846 a rival medical group formed, which then
vowed to slow the development of homeopathy.[19] This organization called itself the American Medical Association.

Members of the AMA had a long-standing animosity toward
homeopathy and homeopaths. This feeling ran so strong that
shortly after the formation of the AMA, it was decided to purge

all the local medical societies of physicians who were homeopaths.[20] This purge was successful in every state except Massachusetts. Because homeopathy was so strong among the elite of Boston, the AMA allowed this exception, so long as the Massachusetts Society agreed not to allow any new homeopathic members. Then, in 1871, the eight remaining homeopathic physicians were expelled from the Society for the heinous crime of being homeopaths.

In 1882, the AMA declined to acknowledge the delegates from the New York State Medical Society because this society had recently passed a resolution that recognized *all* properly graduated doctors (which thereby included homeopathic physicians).

Besides keeping homeopaths out of their societies, the AMA wanted to discourage *any* type of association with homeopaths. In 1855, the AMA established a "consultation clause" within their code of ethics which asserted that orthodox physicians would lose their membership in the AMA if they even consulted with a homeopath or any other "nonregular" practitioner.[21] At the time, if a physician lost his membership in the local medical society, it meant that in some states he no longer had a license to practice medicine. Often, orthodox physicians, who controlled the medical societies, would not admit homeopathic physicians and then would arrange for their arrest for practicing medicine without a license.[22] Ultimately, homeopaths set up their own local societies and established their own medical boards.

At a time in American medicine when physicians were very rarely, if ever, reprimanded by their fellow physicians, the ethical code on consorting with homeopaths was regularly enforced.[23] One Connecticut physician was expelled from his local medical society for consulting with a homeopath—his wife.[24] A New York doctor was expelled for purchasing milk sugar from a homeopathic pharmacy.[25] Joseph K. Barnes, the Surgeon General of the United States, was denounced for aiding in the treatment of Secretary of State William Seward on the night that he was stabbed and Lincoln was shot, simply because Seward's personal physician was a homeopath.[26]

In a bizarre event, Dr. Christopher C. Cox was refused admittance into the Medical Society of the District of Columbia because he had served on the D.C. board of health, which had a member who was a homeopath. Dr. D. W. Bliss, a conventional physician and colleague of Dr. Cox, also was expelled, not because he consulted a homeopath, but because he consulted with Dr. Cox, who was previously expelled. Ironically, the Medical Society judged that Bliss and Cox had committed a heinous crime, even though it was in the treatment of Schulyer Colfax, the Vice President of the United States under Andrew Johnson.[27]

The AMA and its members did everything possible to thwart the education of homeopaths. In the early 1840s and again in 1855, advocates of homeopathy convinced the Michigan legislature to establish a professorship of homeopathy in the department of medicine at the University of Michigan. The AMA resolved to deny recognition to the university's "regular" medical graduates if a homeopath, as one of their professors, signed their diploma (at the time, all professors signed graduates' diplomas). The homeopaths brought their case to the Michigan Supreme Court three times, but each time the court expressed uncertainty as to its power to compel the Regents of the University to take action.[28] Finally, a compromise was reached. In 1875, the Michigan legislature voted to give money to a new hospital as long as two professors of homeopathy were hired to teach at the medical school. It was also decided that only the president and the secretary of the university would sign the diplomas, thereby allowing the graduates to be recognized by the AMA. Despite this compromise, almost every medical journal in the country urged the Michigan medical faculty to resign rather than participate in the training of homeopaths.[29]

The antagonism to homeopathy was not confined only to the United States; it was also widespread in Europe. A French medical student was expelled from his college for expressing interest in homeopathy. A "consultation clause" similar to the one in the United States was established in France. When J. P. Tessier, a conventional French physician, evaluated the results of homeopathy at Hospital Ste. Marguerite and announced to the Paris Academy that they were favorable, he aroused a storm of protest.[30] No orthodox medical journal would publish these results, and when he had it published in a homeopathic journal, he was summarily expelled by the medical society.[31]

In the 1830s, the practice of homeopathy became illegal in

Austria. Despite its illegality, many people used microdoses during the cholera epidemic of 1831. Statistics show that those with cholera who tried homeopathy had a mortality rate between 2.4 and 21.1 percent, whereas over 50 percent of those with cholera under conventional medical care died.[32]

In addition to the attacks by conventional physicians on the homeopaths' right to practice, to join medical organizations, and to gain a medical education, conventional physicians sought to besmirch the reputation of homeopaths. Homeopaths were considered "immoral," "illegitimate," and "unmanly." The opposition to homeopathy was not based on scientific evaluation of this healing art, but arose primarily because homeopaths were significant competitors for conventional physicians.

The Rise of Homeopathy

In an 1890 issue of *Harpers Magazine*, Mark Twain acknowledged the special value of homeopathy, noting: "The introduction of homeopathy forced the old school doctor to stir around and learn something of a rational nature about his business."[33] Twain also asserted that "you may honestly feel grateful that homeopathy survived the attempts of the allopathists [orthodox physicians] to destroy it."

Despite the significant oppression from the orthodox medical profession, homeopathy survived and even thrived in the 1800s and early 1900s. By 1900, there were 22 homeopathic medical schools, more than 100 homeopathic hospitals, over 60 orphan asylums and old people's homes, and more than 1,000 homeopathic pharmacies in the United States.[34] These impressive numbers alone do not provide an accurate perspective on the significant impact that homeopathy had on American life.

Homeopathy attracted support from many of the most respected members of society. Its advocates included William James, Henry Wadsworth Longfellow, Nathaniel Hawthorne, Harriet Beecher Stowe, Daniel Webster, William Seward, Horace Greeley, and Louisa May Alcott. William Cullen Bryant, the famous journalist, was president of the New York Homeopathic Society.[35] John D. Rockefeller referred to homeopathy as "a progressive and aggressive step in medicine." The fact that he was under homeopathic care throughout the latter part of his life may be one reason he lived 99 years.[36]

Homeopathy's popularity among respected classes was also evident in Europe. Besides its patronage by Britain's Royal Family dating from the 1830s,[37] homeopathy could count among its supporters Charles Dickens, W. B. Yeats, William Thackeray, Benjamin Disraeli, Johann Wolfgang Goethe, and Pope Pius X.[38]

Because abolitionists William Lloyd Garrison and Zabina Eastman were strong proponents of homeopathy, and also because many individual homeopaths were politically progressive, homeopathy became identified with the causes of female and black emancipation.[39] Perhaps this spurred homeopathy's popularity in the north,* while retarding its progress in the south.[40]

Homeopathy was also disproportionately popular among women, not only as patients but as its practitioners. The first women's medical college in the world was the homeopathic Boston Female Medical College, founded in 1848. Four years later, it became the New England Female Medical College; and in 1873, it merged with Boston University, another homeopathic college.[41] Homeopaths also admitted women physicians into their national organization considerably before orthodox physicians did. Homeopaths admitted women into the American Institute of Homeopathy in 1871, while women were not invited into the AMA until 1915.[42] The orthodox medical school at Johns Hopkins University finally agreed to accept women students as late as 1890, but not out of an interest in women's rights. It was offered a $500,000 endowment.[43] Harvard University had earlier turned down this same offer.[44]

Many clergy not only were personally supportive of homeopathy but also helped spread the word about it.[45] Even Mary Baker Eddy, the founder of Christian Science, who generally was vehemently opposed to the use of drugs, acknowledged homeopathy's value, saying: "Evidences of progress and of spiritualization greet

---

*Statistics indicate that the number of homeopaths in New York State doubled every five years from 1829 to 1869. (*New England Medical Gazette*, 1869, p. 63.)

us on every hand. Drug-systems are quitting their hold on matter and so letting in matter's higher stratum, mortal mind. Homeopathy, a step in advance of allopathy,* is doing this."[46]

The press was often very supportive of homeopathy, as the *Journal of the American Medical Association* regretfully acknowledged: "We all know perfectly well that the sympathy of the press generally and of the public is with the homeopaths."[47]

It is no wonder that Henry James, another advocate of homeopathy, portrayed this medical science in such a positive light in his novel *The Bostonians.* This reference is carried over in the recent movie made from this book. In a scene from the movie, which is set in the 1880s, Basil Ransom (played by Christopher Reeve) addresses Miss Birdseye, the grand dame of the women's movement (played by Jessica Tandy), as follows:

> Ransom: You must tell me how much you take. One spoonful?
> Birdseye: I guess this time, I'll take two. It's homeopathic.
> Ransom: Oh, I have no doubt of that. I presume you wouldn't have anything else.
> Birdseye: Well, it's generally admitted now to be the true system.[48]

Although homeopathy was particularly popular among the educated and upper classes, it also had a good reputation among the poor. Some of this support no doubt resulted from the free homeopathic dispensaries in many cities.[49]

However, probably the most important reason that homeopathy developed such immense popularity was its success in treating the various epidemic diseases that raged throughout America and Europe during the 1800s. Statistics indicate that the death rates in homeopathic hospitals from these epidemics were often one-half to as little as one-eighth those in orthodox medical hospitals.[50] The homeopaths in Cincinnati were so successful in treating people during the 1849 cholera epidemic that they published a daily list of their patients in the newspaper, giving names and addresses

---

*Allopathy is a word coined by Hahnemann to refer to orthodox medicine.

of those who were cured and those who died. Only 3 percent of the 1,116 homeopathic patients died, while between 48 and 60 percent of those under orthodox medical treatment died.[51]

The success of homeopaths in treating the yellow fever epidemic of 1878 that spread throughout the south was so impressive that homeopathy finally began to be noticed in the region. Death rates for those under homeopathic care were approximately one-third what they were for those using orthodox medicine.[52]

Besides offering effective treatment for infectious diseases, homeopaths provided care for a wide range of acute and chronic disease. The observation that patients under homeopathic care lived longer than others led some life insurance companies to offer a 10 percent discount to homeopathic patients.[53] There is also actuarial evidence that more life insurance money was paid to beneficiaries of homeopathic patients because these people lived longer.[54]

The training of 19th-century homeopaths compared favorably with that of their orthodox physician colleagues. As was mentioned earlier, many homeopaths attended orthodox medical schools. Eventually, homeopaths developed their own medical schools or maintained departments of homeopathy within other medical schools. Boston University, the University of Michigan, the University of Minnesota, Hahnemann Medical College, and the University of Iowa were just a few of the schools teaching homeopathy. Historians today consider the education offered at the homeopathic medical colleges on a par with the orthodox medical schools of the day.[55]

It is impressive to note that a higher percentage of homeopathic medical students passed medical board examinations than did their orthodox medical student colleagues.[56]

Homeopaths showed impressive scholarship, both in books and journals. According to a U.S. Commission on Education in 1898, three of the four medical schools with the largest libraries were homeopathic colleges.[57] And at the turn of the century, there were as many as 29 different homeopathic journals.

Homeopathy's popularity in the United States was obvious and deep-seated. And yet, when reading most books on the history of American medicine, we find little or no mention of it. When there *is* reference, it is generally derogatory, dismissing homeopathy as an anomaly in medicine, a cult that ultimately disappeared, a science of placebos rather than "real drugs," or a medical heresy. It has been said that history is written by the victors, not by the defeated. The history of American medicine is yet another sorry example of this maxim.

The Fall of Homeopathy

It is quite remarkable that homeopathy survived the incessant and harsh attempts to destroy it. After the turn of the century, however, the AMA became increasingly effective in suppressing homeopathy. In a strategic move to make themselves look like "good guys," the AMA chose to "allow" graduates of homeopathic medical schools to join the AMA—so long as they denounced homeopathy or at least did not practice it.[58] The AMA also chose to drop the consultation clause in 1901, not because they were no longer antagonistic to homeopathy, but because they had new efficient ways of defeating it.

In 1910, the Carnegie Foundation issued the infamous Flexner Report, an evaluation of American medical schools chaired by Abraham Flexner in cooperation with leading members of the AMA.[59] While pretending to be objective, the report actually established guidelines meant to sanction orthodox medical schools and condemn homeopathic ones. The report placed the highest value on those medical schools that had a full-time teaching faculty and taught a pathological and physiochemical analysis of the human body. Homeopathic colleges were faulted because of their preference for employing professors who were not simply teachers or researchers but also in clinical practice. Although homeopathic schools included many basic science courses, they also had courses in pharmacology, which the Flexner Report did not consider worthwhile.

As one might easily predict, the homeopathic colleges on the whole were given poor ratings by the Flexner Report. As a result of the report, only graduates of those schools that received a high rating were allowed to take medical licensing exams. There were twenty-two homeopathic colleges in 1900, but only two remained by 1923.[60]

These schools were not the only ones hurt by the Flexner Report. Of the seven black medical schools, only two survived. The report also contributed to a 33 percent reduction in women graduates from medical schools.[61]

As a way of coping with new guidelines and in order to pass the new licensing exams that stressed the basic sciences, homeopathic colleges decided to offer more education on pathology, chemistry, physiology, and other medical sciences. However, although they offered better education on these subjects, their homeopathic training suffered greatly.[62] As a result, the graduates from these homeopathic colleges were less able to practice homeopathy well. Instead of individualizing medicines to a person's totality of symptoms, many homeopaths began prescribing medicines according to disease categories. The consequences of this type of care was predictably poor. Many homeopaths gave up homeopathic practice, and many homeopathic patients sought other types of care.

There were other reasons for the sharp decline of homeopathy after the turn of the century. Orthodox medicine was no longer as barbaric as it had been in the 1800s, and because of this it did not drive as many patients away. Orthodox physicians also began incorporating several of the homeopathic medicines into their practice. Although they did not prescribe the same small doses as the homeopaths, their use of certain homeopathic medicines confused the public, who were having increasing difficulty in distinguishing orthodox from homeopathic physicians.[63]

Another factor in the decline of homeopathy was its economic viability. Good homeopathic practice required individualization of the patient, which demanded more time than most orthodox physicians gave to their patients. Since economics governs the way medicine is practiced more than is commonly recognized, the fact that physicians in the 20th century could make more money practicing orthodox medicine is a significant factor that led to homeopathy's decline.

Perhaps history could have been changed if John D. Rockefeller, a strong advocate of homeopathy, had given the major grants he intended to homeopathic institutions. He had instructed his financial adviser, Frederick Gates, to do so. Since Gates was totally partial to orthodox medicine, he never complied with Rockefeller's orders.[64] This loss of potential funding was tragic, since Rockefeller gave away between $300 and $400 million in the early 1900s, most of which went to orthodox medical institutions.[65]

The drug companies' antagonism to homeopathy contributed significantly to the collective efforts to suppress this form of medicine. Because the drug companies published medical journals, they could use them as mouthpieces against homeopathy and in support of orthodox medicine. Even an article in a 1906 issue of the *Journal of the American Medical Association* acknowledged that "the medical press is profoundly under the influence of the proprietary interests [drug companies]."[66]

Along with the various external factors that hindered homeopathy's growth, there were problems among homeopaths themselves. Disagreement within homeopathy has a long tradition. Hahnemann demanded that his followers practice precisely the way he did: "He who does not walk on exactly the same line with me, who diverges, if it be but the breadth of a straw, to the right or to the left, is an apostate and a traitor."[67] As one could predict, many homeopaths did not practice as Hahnemann did.

The most famous homeopaths in the United States were primarily Hahnemannians. However, the majority of homeopaths practicing in this country did not prescribe their medicines on the basis of the totality of symptoms, but primarily according to the chief complaint. These homeopaths prescribed medicines for specific diseases, and sometimes they prescribed one medicine for a person's headache, another for his digestive disorder, and yet another for his skin problem. Hahnemann and his followers were particularly adamant about the use of only one medicine at a time, and Hahnemann referred to those practitioners who used more than a single medicine as "pseudo-homeopaths" or worse.

Throughout his life, Hahnemann primarily used medicines that were potentized 3, 6, 9, 12, or 30 times. Toward the end of his life, however, some of his colleagues experimented successfully with medicines that had been potentized 90, 200, 1,000, or 10,000 times. In 1829, Hahnemann wrote a letter to a friend, expressing disbelief in the effectiveness of these medicines. He was also concerned that the public would not place trust in homeopathy if prac titioners utilized such extremely dilute medicines. He recommended that homeopaths not use anything more dilute than the 30th potency.[68] Later, Hahnemann acknowledged that these higher potencies had effect, though there is no record of him ever using a medicine higher than the 1,500th potency.*

After Hahnemann's death, the vast majority of Hahnemannian homeopaths adopted the higher potencies. The low-potency homeopaths, however, were not converted, and the stage was set for yet another opportunity for disagreement among homeopaths. The high- and low-potency schools of thought developed separate organizations, hospitals, and journals. In 1901, because of the various diagreements among homeopaths, Chicago had four different homeopathic medical societies.

The poor training that the homeopathic schools offered after the turn of the century ultimately discouraged the rigorous approach that the Hahnemann method required.

From 1930 to 1975, there were not many horror stories about the AMA's oppression of homeopathy, primarily because it seemed that the AMA had already won the war. By 1950, all the homeopathic colleges in the United States were either closed or no longer teaching homeopathy. There were only 50 to 150 practicing homeopathic physicians, and most of these were over 50 years old.

And yet, it is hard to suppress the truth. Homeopathy has risen again, and this time history will be rewritten.

The Present Status of Homeopathy

Homeopaths in other countries have experienced varying degrees of opposition from orthodox physicians, but not anywhere near the systematic and intense attacks suffered by American homeopaths at the hands of American doctors. When homeopaths have been given a relatively free environment to practice, homeopathy has been able to grow and flourish.

Homeopathy is particularly popular in Great Britain, where,

---

*Higher-potency medicines are those that have been potentized 200, 1,000, 10,000, 100,000, or more times; lower potencies are potentized 3, 6, 9, or 12 times; a medium potency is one potentized 30 times.

as already noted, the Royal Family has been under homeopathic care since the 1830s.[69] The *New York Times* noted that visits to homeopathic physicians are increasing in England at a rate of 39 percent per year.[70] A British consumer organization surveyed its 28,000 members and discovered that 80 percent had used some form of complementary medicine* and that 70 percent of those who had tried homeopathy were cured or improved by it.[71] Not only is there growing interest from the general public, but there is also surprising acknowledgment of homeopathy by conventional physicians. The *British Medical Journal* recently published a survey of the attitudes of British physicians toward practitioners of complementary medicine. The survey discovered that 42 percent of the physicians surveyed refer patients to homeopathic physicians.[72] A different study published in the *Times* of London found that 48 percent of physicians referred patients to homeopathic physicians.[73] A study published in the *British Medical Journal* noted that in a survey of 100 recently graduated British physicians, 80 percent expressed an interest in being trained in either homeopathy, acupuncture, or hypnosis.[74]

This impressive growth in Great Britain is being matched in France. A recent survey of French doctors revealed that approximately 11,000 utilize homeopathic medicines, approximately 25 percent of the French public have tried or are presently using homeopathic medicines, and over 20,000 French pharmacies now sell homeopathic medicines.[75] This survey also noted that courses in homeopathy leading to a degree are offered in six medical schools. Homeopathy is taught in all pharmacy schools and in four veterinary schools. Homeopathy is growing so rapidly in France that a recent cover story of *Le Nouvel Observateur*, one of France's leading magazines, noted that President Mitterrand and six medical school deans had called for more research on homeopathy.[76] The author editorialized: "It is a fact that homeopathy obtains results,

---

*In Great Britain and to a small extent in the United States, "complementary medicine" or "complementary therapies" are replacing the terms "alternative medicine" or "alternative therapies." Advocates of complementary therapies assert that their therapies are not "alternative" but are a growing part of mainstream medicine.

sometimes spectacular results."

In 1981, the Dutch government published a report on *Alternative Medicine in The Netherlands,* which concluded that 20 percent of the Dutch public utilize alternative healing methods. The report also noted that homeopathy is one of the most popular therapeutic modalities.[77]

Homeopathy is widespread in Europe, but it is even more popular in Asia, especially India, Pakistan, and Sri Lanka. Homeopathy spread like wildfire in India, in part because of the support it received from Mahatma Gandhi, but also because it has been effective in treating many of the acute infectious conditions and chronic maladies on the subcontinent. As an article in the World Health Organization's journal *World Health Forum* noted: "Homeopathic treatment seems well suited for use in rural areas where the infrastructure, equipment, and drugs needed for conventional medicine cannot be provided."[78] Homeopathy is also considerably cheaper than conventional medicine, and any person, not just physicians, can learn to use a small number of medicines for simple common complaints.

Presently, there are over 120 four- or five-year homeopathic medical schools in India. Nineteen of the colleges are maintained by the state, most of which are affiliated with universities.[79] It has been estimated that there are over 100,000 homeopathic practitioners in India. An article in the *World Health Forum* acknowledged that "in the Indian subcontinent the legal position of the practitioners of homeopathy has been elevated to a professional level similar to that of a medical practitioner."[80]

Homeopathy is not as popular in South America as it is in Europe or Asia, but it is still widely utilized. Homeopathy's popularity in Argentina dates back to General San Martín, the country's greatest hero, who was reported to have taken a kit of homeopathic medicines across the Andes in his efforts to free Chile and Peru from Spain in 1816. One of Argentina's most respected homeopathic physicians, Dr. Francisco Eizayaga, has estimated that there are now approximately 2,000 doctors in Argentina who practice homeopathy and approximately 3 million people who have used homeopathic medicines.[81]

Homeopathy is equally popular in Brazil, where there are

also approximately 2,000 physicians who utilize homeopathic medicines. It is interesting to note that pharmacists in Brazil are required to take a course in homeopathic pharmacology in order to graduate. There are at least ten homeopathic schools in Brazil, and several conventional medical schools have coursework in homeopathy.[82]

Besides homeopathy's special popularity in the previously mentioned countries, it is also widely practiced in Mexico, Greece, Belgium, Italy, Spain, Australia, South Africa, Nigeria, and the Soviet Union.

Homeopathy is reexperiencing a renaissance in the United States as well. In the early 1970s, there were only 50 to 100 physicians who specialized in homeopathy, and yet by the mid-1980s, it can be estimated that there are approximately 1,000 physicians who specialize in homeopathy. According to the *Washington Post,* the numbers of physicians in the United States who specialize in homeopathy doubled from 1980 to 1982.[83]

There is a concomitant increase in the use of microdoses by various other health professionals. Approximately 1,000 other health professionals in the United States use homeopathic medicines, and these include dentists, podiatrists, veterinarians, physician assistants, nurses, naturopaths, acupuncturists, chiropractors, and psychologists. Although these numbers still represent only a very small percentage of licensed health professionals, the rapidly growing interest in homeopathy portends significant increases to come.

The rediscovery of homeopathy by the general public is even more encouraging. The magazine *FDA Consumer* recently reported a 1000 percent increase in sales of homeopathic medicines from the late 1970s to the early 1980s.[84]

Contrary to some critics who think that people try homeopathy only because they are uneducated, research published in the *Western Journal of Medicine* shows that homeopathic patients tend to be better educated than the average American.[85]

It is difficult to predict how popular homeopathy will be in the United States in the 21st century, though it is probable that most physicians will utilize at least some of the microdoses that research has proven to be effective. Growing numbers of consumers will also learn to self-prescribe homeopathic medicine for common acute conditions and will probably demand homeopathic care from their physicians for more serious medical conditions.

Clearly, homeopathy will play an increasingly important role in health care, for as internationally acclaimed violinist and humanitarian Yehudi Menuhin once said: "Homeopathy is one of the few medical specialties which carries no penalties—only benefits."

Notes

1. Sir James George Frazer, *The Golden Bough* (New York: Macmillan, 1922), pp. 12–42.

2. Richard Haehl, *Samuel Hahnemann: His Life and Work* (New Delhi: B. Jain, 1971), p. 37.

3. Trevor M. Cook, *Samuel Hahnemann: The Founder of Homoeopathic Medicine* (Wellingborough, England: Thorsons, 1981), pp. 71–77; Harris L. Coulter, *Divided Legacy* (Washington, D.C.: Wehawken, 1977), vol. 2, p. 310.

4. Samuel Hahnemann, "Essay on a New Principle for Ascertaining the Curative Powers of Drugs, and Some Examinations of the Previous Principles," *Hufeland's Journal*, 2 (1796): 391–439, 465–561.

5. Thomas L. Bradford, *The Life and Letters of Dr. Samuel Hahnemann* (Philadelphia: Boericke and Tafel, 1895), p. 151.

6. Cook, *Samuel Hahnemann*, p. 127.

7. Haehl, *Samuel Hahnemann*, p. 108.

8. Cook, *Samuel Hahnemann*, p. 130.

9. Paul Starr, *The Social Transformation of American Medicine* (New York: Basic, 1982).

10. Cook, *Samuel Hahnemann*, p. 39.

11. Harris L. Coulter, *Divided Legacy* (Berkeley: North Atlantic Books, 1975), vol. 3, p. 39.

12. Cook, *Samuel Hahnemann*, p. 39.

13. Coulter, *Divided Legacy*, vol. 3, p. 70

14. *New York Journal of Medicine*, 5 (1845): 418.

15. Coulter, *Divided Legacy*, vol. 3, p. 103.

16. Starr, *Social Transformation*, p. 97.

17. Martin Kaufman, *Homoeopathy in America* (Baltimore: Johns Hopkins University Press, 1971), p. 158.

18. Coulter, *Divided Legacy*, vol. 3, pp. 124–126.

19. Kaufman, *Homoeopathy in America*, p. 53.

20. Coulter, *Divided Legacy*, vol. 3, p. 199.

21. Ibid., pp. 206–219.

22. William Harvey King, *History of Homeopathy* (New York: Lewis, 1905), vol. 1, p. 47.

23. Coulter, *Divided Legacy*, vol. 3, p. 208.

24. Starr, *Social Transformation*, p. 98.

25. Ibid.

26. Ibid.

27. Kaufman, *Homeopathy in America*, p. 89.

28. Coulter, *Divided Legacy*, vol. 3, p. 208.

29. Ibid., 209.

30. Bradford, *Dr. Samuel Hahnemann*, p. 157.

31. Coulter, *Divided Legacy*, vol. 3, p. 562.

32. Cook, *Samuel Hahnemann*, p. 158; Thomas L. Bradford, *The Logic of Figures or Comparative Results of Homoeopathic and Other Treatments* (Philadelphia: Boericke and Tafel, 1900), pp. 112–146.

33. Mark Twain, "A Majestic Literary Fossil," *Harpers Magazine*, February 1890, p. 444.

34. Coulter, *Divided Legacy*, vol. 3, pp. 304, 460; *Transactions of the American Institute of Homoeopathy*, 1901, pp. 657–746.

35. King, *History of Homeopathy*, vol. 2, p. 14.

36. Coulter, *Divided Legacy*, vol. 3, p. 463.

37. Cook, *Samuel Hahnemann*, pp. 142–144.

38. Ibid., p. 148; *New England Medical Gazette*, 1869, p. 291; *Transaction of the American Institute of Homoeopathy*, 1908, p. 128.

39. King, *History of Homeopathy*, vol. 1, p. 346.

40. Coulter, *Divided Legacy*, vol. 3, p. 297.

41. King, *History of Homeopathy*, vol. 2, pp. 159–213.

42. Ruth Abrams, ed., *Send Us a Lady Physician: Women Doctors in America, 1835–1920* (New York: Norton, 1985), p. 100.

43. Starr, *Social Transformation*, p. 117.

44. Abrams, ed., *Lady Physician*, p. 101.

45. Coulter, *Divided Legacy*, vol. 3, p. 112.

46. Mary Baker Eddy, *Science and Health*.

47. *Transactions of the Medical Society of the State of New York*, 1872, p. 46.

48. Henry James, *The Bostonians* (New York: Bantam, 1984), p. 315.

49. Coulter, *Divided Legacy*, vol. 3, p. 113.

50. Bradford, *Logic of Figures*, p. 59; Coulter, *Divided Legacy*, vol. 3, pp. 298–305.

51. Bradford, *Logic of Figures*, pp. 68, 113–146; Coulter, *Divided Legacy*, vol. 3, p. 268.

52. Coulter, *Divided Legacy*, vol. 3, pp. 299–302.

53. *New England Medical Gazette*, 1866, p. 69.

54. *Transactions of the American Institute of Homoeopathy*, 1892, p. 83.

55. Kaufman, *Homoeopathy in America*, p. 58.

56. *Transactions of the American Institute of Homoeopathy*, 1893, p. 52; *Journal of the American Medical Association*, 52 (May 22, 1909): 1691ff.

57. *Phials*, University of Michigan, 1901.

58. Coulter, *Divided Legacy*, vol. 3, p. 430.

59. Starr, *Social Transformation*, p. 119; Coulter, *Divided Legacy*, vol. 3, p. 446.

60. Kaufman, *Homoeopathy in America*, p. 166.

61. Starr, *Social Transformation*, p. 124.

62. Coulter, *Divided Legacy*, vol. 3, p. 444.

63. Ibid., p. 371.

64. E. Richard Brown, *Rockefeller's Medicine Men* (Berkeley: University of California Press, 1979), pp. 109–111.

65. Ibid.

66. J. H. Salisbury, "The Subordination of Medical Journals to Proprietary Interests," *Journal of the American Medical Association*, 46 (1906): 1337–38.

67. Bradford, *Dr. Samuel Hahnemann*, p. 304.

68. Ibid., pp. 455–456.

69. Trevor Cook, *Samuel Hahnemann: The Founder of Homoeopathic Medicine* (Wellingborough, England: Thorsons, 1981), p. 144.

70. Barnaby J. Feder, "Holistic Medicine in Britain," *New York Times*, January 9, 1985.

71. "Magic or Medicine," *Which?* October 1986, pp. 443–447.

72. Richard Wharton and George Lewith, "Complementary Medicine and the General Practitioner," *British Medical Journal*, 292 (June 7, 1986): 1498–1500.

73. "Taking the Alternative Path to Health," *Times* (London), March 13, 1985.

74. David Taylor Reilly, "Young Doctors' Views on Alternative Medicine," *British Medical Journal*, 287 (July 30, 1983): 337–339.

75. IFOP Survey, Paris, 1985.

76. "Médecines douches: La revanche de l'homéopathie," *Le Nouvel Observateur*, April 12, 1985, pp. 36–41.

77. "Summary Report of the Commission for Alternative Systems of Medicine," *Alternative Medicine in The Netherlands*, The Hague, 1981, pp. 10–11.

78. Jugal Kishore, "Homoeopathy: The Indian Experience," *World Health Forum*, 3 (1983): 107.

79. Ibid., p. 106.

80. Ibid., p. 110.

81. Francisco X. Eizayaga, "Homeopathy in American Spanish-Speaking Countries," A Presentation at the Annual Conference of the National Center for Homeopathy, October 4–5, 1985.

82. *World Homoeopathic Directory* (New Delhi: Harjeet, 1982), pp. 36–37; Eizayaga, "Homeopathy."

83. Ann Chase, "Options: Homeopathy," *Washington Post*, April 28, 1983, p. D5.

84. "Riding the Coattails of Homeopathy," *FDA Consumer*, March 1985, p. 31.

85. R. L. Avina and L. J. Schneiderman, "Why Patients Choose Homeopathy," *Western Journal of Medicine*, 128 (April 1978): 366–369.

3

Homeopathic Research: Scientific Verification of Homeopathic Medicine

Even Sir William Osler, considered to be the father of modern medicine, acknowledged the homeopaths' serious interest in scientific medicine. Speaking to a group of conventional physicians in 1905, Osler stated: "It is not as if our homeopathic brothers are asleep: far from it, they are awake—many of them at any rate—to the importance of the scientific study of disease."[1]

When skeptics today say that there is no research on homeopathy, it is because they have not kept up-to-date on the latest developments in science and medicine; there are, in fact, dozens of good scientific studies on homeopathy. More research is indeed essential for us to learn more about homeopathy, but no one should ignore the scientific investigation that has already been done on this pharmacological method.

Skeptics sometimes assume that the microdoses that homeopaths use could not possibly have any biological or clinical effects. Even when confirming research on homeopathy is published in respected scientific journals, many conventional physicians will deny the possibility that the medicines actually worked. Some physicians recently ridiculed some double-blind* homeopathic

---

*A double-blind experiment is one in which the researchers and the subjects of the experiment do not know which subjects are receiving the treatment being tested and which are receiving a placebo.

research published in the prestigious medical journal *Lancet* by suggesting that the researchers were testing one placebo versus another.[2] The authors of the research replied to this response by expressing concern at their critics' nihilistic view of the scientific method, since the double-blind methodology is widely recognized as an accepted way to distinguish placebo responses from the actions of medicines.[3]

Although some skeptics are closed-minded to homeopathy and do not want to be confused by the facts, there are a growing number of physicians and scientists who acknowledge that careful research has demonstrated the action of the homeopathic medicines. They now seek to understand its implications.

Still other people do not care if homeopathy can be explained or if research has "proven" it or not. These people may have experienced the value of the medicines in the past, and they are only interested in knowing if it can work for them in the future. They are more persuaded by their own experience than by what someone else defines as "scientific."

The Empirical Evidence

Whether one is or is not convinced by or interested in homeopathic research, it is worthwhile to note the following facts, which suggest that the homeopathic medicines are not placebos and that the doses used have biological action.

1. *Homeopathic medicines are commonly used on animals by veterinarians and laypersons.* The successful experience of treating animals with microdoses has been significant enough that entire books have been written on the homeopathic treatment of dogs, cats, horses, and even cattle. There have also been some significant double-blind clinical studies on animals (discussed below in the section "Clinical Trials on Animals"). Although a certain degree of suggestion may be possible with animals, it seems doubtful that mere psychological support could be significant enough to cure a dog's neurological condition, a cat's abscess, a horse's skin problem, or a cow's mastitis with the kind of consistency experienced by those who use the homeopathic medicine. It is more likely that the medicines

themselves have an effect and are not acting only as placebos.

2. *Homeopathic medicines are commonly used on infants.* Infants also may be somewhat suggestible, but it is common for homeopaths and parents to observe almost immediate effects of homeopathic medicines on infants' teething difficulties, feverish conditions, sleepless states, and neurological disorders. Explaining these effects simply as the results of placebos is inadequate. (See Chapter 5 on pediatrics for more information on the homeopathic treatment of infants and children.)

3. *Homeopathy became particularly popular in the United States and Europe in the 1800s because of its success in treating the epidemics that raged during that time, including cholera, typhoid, yellow fever, and scarlet fever.* It is again doubtful that placebos could have been very effective in treating these serious infectious diseases.

4. *The homeopathic medicines have the capacity to heal when they are prescribed in the proper microdose, but they also have the capacity to create the symptoms they are known to heal if certain sensitive people recurrently take microdoses of that particular substance.* The primary way that homeopaths discover what group of symptoms a medicine can treat effectively is to conduct experiments called "provings." Small doses of a substance are given once or twice a day for several weeks until those persons sensitive to the substance develop symptoms. These doses may be 3x, 6x, or 9x of the medicine being tested (all of which have a very small but measurable amount of the substance). At other times the provings are done with 30x, 200x, or higher (more dilute) potencies. The concentration of the original substance in these doses is so small that in all probability there are not any remaining molecules of the substance being tested. And yet, when taken continually, each medicine has the capacity to cause its own unique set of symptoms.

The fact that the homeopathic microdoses have the capacity not only to heal but also to cause symptoms provides some evidence that highly dilute medicines have biological action. It is indeed rare for a placebo to cause a similar group of symptoms in people, and thus one can assume that the microdoses are *not* placebos.

5. *When a person with a chronic illness is given a homeopathic medicine, it is relatively common for that person to experience "a healing crisis"—that is, a temporary exacerbation of symptoms that he presently has or may have had in the past.* Placebos generally cause no reaction, though they can effectively alleviate symptoms at times, and less often they can cause an aggravation of symptoms. Since homeopaths who use high-potency medicines (those in the 200th, 1,000th, 10,000th, or 50,000th potency) observe a healing crisis in 10 to 30 percent of their patients, it is unlikely that a placebo can be the sole cause.

6. *Presently, many homeopathic pharmacies in the United States voluntarily restrict the use of the higher potencies (200th, 1,000th, 10,000th, and higher) to licensed health professionals.* Although selling the high potencies to the general public might be financially beneficial to the pharmacies, they respect the power of the higher potencies and thus restrict their availability. Now that the public is receiving more education on how to use homeopathic medicines, some pharmacies are no longer restricting over-the-counter sales.

In the light of the above six empirical observations, there is already a strong *prima facie* case for the action of the homeopathic microdoses. But in addition to such empirical evidence, several double-blind experiments provide significant further support for the biological action and the clinical efficiency of the homeopathic pharmaceuticals.

Clinical Evidence

Conducting clinical research is considerably more difficult than one might initially suppose. Despite all the money and manpower devoted to assessing conventional medical treatments, a report on the efficacy of all medical care issued by the U.S. Congress's Office of Technology Assessment concluded by stating, "It has been estimated that only 10 to 20 percent of all procedures currently used in medical practice have been shown to be efficacious by controlled trial."[4]

There are even more limited funds available for homeopathic research, but the studies of efficacy are at least as convincing as those carried out on other medical procedures.

One of the first double-blind experiments ever performed was sponsored by a homeopathic organization in 1906. This experiment was a proving of *Belladonna* (deadly nightshade) and was conducted in eleven cities with a total of fifty-one subjects. An impressive mass of symptoms was collected from these subjects, most of which confirmed what was previously known about the toxicity of *Belladonna*.[5]

Another early double-blind study was sponsored by the British government during World War II. The experiment showed that those subjects given *Mustard gas 30c*, * *Rhus tox 30c* (poison ivy), or *Kali bichromicum 30c* (bichromate of potash) experienced significant improvement in burns from mustard gas in comparison to those given a placebo.[6] A recent analysis of this study provided further substantiation of the statistical significance of this research.[7]

A double-blind trial of the homeopathic treatment of patients with hay fever was recently published in *Lancet*.[8] This study was conducted by two representatives of the Glasgow Homeopathic Hospital and was independently evaluated by representatives of the University of Glasgow's departments of statistics and immunology. The study compared hay fever patients who were given a homeopathic preparation of twelve mixed pollens in the 30c dose with hay fever patients given a placebo. The study showed that those given a homeopathic medicine had six times fewer symptoms than those given a placebo. Both groups of patients were allowed to take an antihistamine if their symptoms warranted it. By the end of the study, those given the homeopathic medicine chose to take this conventional drug *half* as often as did those given a placebo.

A double-blind experiment on patients with rheumatoid arthritis was published in the *British Journal of Clinical Pharmacology*.[9] Each patient was individually prescribed a homeopathic medicine, but only half were given this homeopathic medicine,

---

*The letter *c* after a number refers to the serial dilution 1:99; the letter *x* after a number refers to the serial dilution 1:9.

while the other half were given a placebo. The results showed that an impressive 82 percent of those given a homeopathic medicine experienced some relief of symptoms, while only 21 percent of those given a placebo experienced a similar degree of improvement.

A uniquely designed double-blind experiment was conducted on patients suffering from fibrositis, a rheumatological disease.[10] The research design allowed the homeopaths to prescribe one of only three medicines (*Arnica*, *Rhus tox*, and *Bryonia*—mountain daisy, poison ivy, and wild hops, respectively). There was no statistical difference between the group given a homeopathic medicine and the group given a placebo. However, as part of the research design, the accuracy of the prescription itself was evaluated by a panel of homeopathic physicians. This secondary evaluation showed that there *was* a statistically significant difference between those subjects the panel concluded were given the *correct* homeopathic medicine and those given a placebo. (The panel did not know in advance which patients had experienced improvement.) This particular experiment indicates that it is not enough to expect improvement simply from giving a homeopathic medicine; the remedy must be individualized to the sick person.

Another double-blind trial was conducted on patients with dental neuralgic pain following tooth extraction.[11] Thirty patients were given *Arnica 7c* (mountain daisy) and *Hypericum 15c* (St. John's wort), prescribed alternately at four-hour intervals, and thirty other patients were given a placebo. An impressive 76 percent of those given the homeopathic medicines experienced relief of pain, while only 40 percent of those given a placebo experienced similar relief.

Another study, published in a respected German pharmacological journal, showed that a homeopathic combination medicine* was effective in reducing vertigo and nausea.[12] By both subjective and objective measures, those subjects given this medicine had a statistically significant improvement in comparison to those given a placebo.

---

*A combination medicine is one in which more than one remedy is combined in the same pellet or bottle.

French researchers recently completed a double-blind trial using a combination medicine to treat pregnant women. The study found that the homeopathic medicine significantly reduced child-birth time and decreased abnormal labor. Ninety-three women were involved in the experiment; forty were given a placebo and fifty-three were given a 5c combination medicine, which included *Caulophyllum* (blue cohosh), *Actea raemosa* (cimicifuga or black snakeroot), *Arnica* (mountain daisy), *Pulsatilla* (windflower), and *Gelsemium* (yellow jasmine). The researchers found that women given the homeopathic medicine were in labor for an average of 5.1 hours, while those given a placebo were in labor for an average of 8.5 hours. Only 11.3 percent of the women given the homeo-pathic medicine had an abnormal labor, while 40 percent of those given a placebo had an abnormal labor.[13]

One experiment which did not show that the homeopathic medicines were effective should also be mentioned. Patients with osteoarthritis were either given *Rhus tox 6x*, fenoprofen (a con-ventional drug with anti-inflammatory analgesic effects), or a placebo. The study showed that those persons given the conven-tional drug experienced the greatest relief of symptoms. Those given *Rhus tox 6x* did not experience any more improvement than did those given a placebo.[14]

One might initially conclude, if taking this study in isolation, that homeopathic medicines are inactive substances, like placebos. However, homeopaths have responded to this particular experi-ment by noting that a strategy of using only one medicine, rather than individualizing medicines according to the totality of symp-toms, can be effective only in very select conditions.[15] Osteoar-thritis is not one of these. It was clearly inappropriate for *Rhus tox* to be chosen for the treatment of osteoarthritis, since it is not often given for this condition, though it is often prescribed for rheumatoid arthritis. The study design of this trial was further ill-conceived because it inappropriately compared, over a short period of time, a fast-acting drug (the anti-inflammatory analgesic) and a slow-acting one (the homeopathic medicine). A similar ex-periment comparing results in the treatment of pain with mor-phine versus a homeopathic medicine would also show better short-term results with morphine, but this would not necessarily mear that morphine is more curative in the long run than the indicated homeopathic remedy.

Clinical Trials on Animals

Experiments on animals have a special value, since a placebo effect is less likely to be induced. Hence, in the following double-blind trials, one may conclude with relative certainty that the homeopathic medicines being tested did have beneficial action.

One study completed by four German scientists at a veterinary college showed that *Chelidonium 3x* (celandine) lowered serum cholesterol when given twice a day to rabbits on a cholesterol-rich diet.[16] After thirty-four days, the seven rabbits treated with homeopathic medicine displayed about 25 percent lower serum cholesterol concentrations than the seven rabbits given a placebo.

An important study was published in a respected journal, *Human Toxicology*, which showed that microdoses of arsenic helped rats to eliminate crude doses of arsenic that they had been previously fed.[17] This research compared various potencies of *Arsenicum album* (arsenic), including 10x, 14x, 18x, 22x, 26x, 30x, 5c, 7c, 9c, 11c, 13c, and 15c. All these potencies helped the rats to eliminate the arsenic, unlike those rats that were given a placebo. The best results were observed from the 14x and 7c potencies. The research also found that, overall, the "x" potencies augmented elimination of arsenic more than the "c" potencies. Considering that environmental exposure to heavy metals has become a significant problem in this modern world, more research that explores the use of homeopathic medicines in helping to eliminate toxic substances should be of vital importance.

British veterinarian Cristopher Day used *Caulophyllum 30c* (blue cohosh) on pigs that were known to have a high rate of stillbirths.[18] Those pigs given a placebo had 103 births and 27 stillbirths (20.8 percent), while those given the homeopathic medicine had 104 births and 12 stillbirths (10.3 percent).

Christopher Day also conducted several pilot studies which suggested that homeopathic medicine can reduce labor problems in cattle and decrease bovine mastitis.[19]

A researcher at a cancer research center in India found that those mice that received a transplantation of fibrosarcoma (a type of cancer) and then were treated with homeopathic medicines survived significantly longer than untreated mice.[20] Of the 77 mice treated homeopathically, 52 percent survived more than one year, while all 77 untreated mice died within 10–15 days.

Another important experiment on rodents showed that homeopathic medicines must work along recognized biochemical pathways in inhibiting pain response.[21] Scientists at a British school of pharmacy found that rodents given *Hypericum 30c* (St. John's wort) were able to remain on a hot plate longer than those given water. The rodents were tested again with *Hypericum 30c*, and this time they were also given naloxone, a chemical that is known to inhibit the endorphin or pain-killing response. Naloxone was found to reduce the protective effects of *Hypericum*. Since naloxone is also known to reduce the pain-killing response of morphine, the researchers concluded that the homeopathic medicine seemed to be stimulating a similar biochemical action.

Although this research and some of the others mentioned in this section have a special value in demonstrating that microdoses are efficacious and even in hinting toward how they work, it should be noted that many animal studies do not respect the rights of animals. Such research should be kept to a minimum.

Laboratory Evidence

Laboratory research cannot prove or disprove any specific or even general effect of homeopathic medicines on human health; it can only point toward what, if any, biological consequences the microdoses have. Some well-designed research may even give clues toward helping us to understand more difficult questions—*how* and *why* microdoses work.

Nuclear magnetic resonance, or NMR (sometimes called magnetic resonance imaging), is a state-of-the-art medical technology that can measure the spin of protons. A recent NMR study showed that twenty-three different homeopathic medicines and potencies had distinctive readings of subatomic activity, while a placebo did not.[22]

French researchers showed that potentized doses of *Apis*

(crushed bee) and *Histamine* had a statistically significant effect on reducing the release of certain allergy-causing chemicals from basophils (a type of white blood cell that is related to allergy symptoms). This research implies that these medicines may be helpful in reducing the symptoms of allergies.[23]

Some research published in the *International Journal of Immunotherapy* provided evidence that potentized doses of blood (5x, 7x) demonstrated an inhibiting effect on basophil degranulation.[24] This effect was evidenced after exposure to fourteen of eighteen allergens, including tree pollens, mold, mites, house dust, Penicillin, Candida albicans, and aspirin.

Another study published in a respected pharmacology journal showed that *Silica 6c* and *Silica 10c* had statistically significant effects on stimulating macrophages in mice.[25] (Macrophages are essential parts of the immune system and help to destroy foreign particles, bacteria, and other cells.) This evidence showing that homeopathic medicines can be used to stimulate immune responses is of particular importance.

A study showing the antiviral activity of homeopathic medicines may have special importance today because of the sudden global increase in serious viral infections. An experiment on chicken embryos showed that eight out of ten homeopathic medicines tested inhibited viruses between 50 and 100 percent.[26] The researchers also tested four different medicines on a virus that infects mice, but they did not find any benefit from any of them. This experiment, once again, indicates that choosing the correct medicines is essential to receiving the desired effects.

One extensive and meticulously controlled experiment was carried out in 1941 and 1942 by a Scottish homeopath and scientist, W. E. Boyd.[27] Boyd showed that microdoses of mercuric chloride had statistically significant effects on diastase activity (diastase is an enzyme produced during the germination of seeds). An associate dean of an American medical school was so impressed with Dr. Boyd's research that he said that "the precision of [Boyd's] technique exemplifies a scientific study at its highest level."[28]

Boyd's experiment was so well controlled that any present attempt to recreate it would be inordinately expensive. Raynor Jones and Michael Jenkins, two British researchers, recently completed comparable, though easier and less expensive experiments on yeast and wheat seedlings.[29] These tests showed that *Pulsatilla* (windflower) in varying potencies up to 13c caused increased growth of the yeast and wheat seedlings as compared to the effects of distilled water on equivalent organisms.

It should be noted that British researcher William Steffan tried to replicate this experiment but did not get similar results.[30] However, two other researchers reanalyzed Steffan's results and found that Steffan's work had, in fact, confirmed that of Jones and Jenkins.[31]

Although research often requires specialized knowledge in an area of science, some experiments are simple and can be done by anyone who puts his or her mind and time into them. Jessica Chou, a high school student in San Diego, California, completed a science project for her school on homeopathic medicine. She showed that potentized doses of a commercial fertilizer had statistically significant effects on mung seed sprouts. Her scientific methodology and results were so impressive that she won several awards for her project, and her research was published in the *Journal of the American Institute of Homeopathy.*[32]

In addition to the various studies described here which indicate that homeopathic microdoses have biological action and clinical efficacy, A. R. D. Stebbing, a British scientist (not a homeopath), has referenced over 100 studies from various scientific fields which show that microdoses of certain substances can have even greater effects upon a system than larger doses.[33] Although the studies do not make reference to the extreme microdoses utilized in homeopathy, Stebbing does provide important evidence of the power of small doses of certain substances on discrete systems.

Implications of Homeopathic Research

The implications of homeopathic research are profound and difficult to overestimate. Our very understanding of the human organism may become more sophisticated. The fact that homeopathic medicines have any biological action at all encourages us to accept the possibility of a bioenergetic process of the body that apparently is able to receive and act upon these microdoses. Greater understanding of this bioenergetic process may provide science with some of the missing links of physiological function that presently elude researchers. Some of the mysteries of the body await being unlocked upon scientific investigation of this underlying interconnective force.

The implications of homeopathic research encourage us to investigate not only when and how the medicines can be used in treating human ills, but when and how they can be applied to problems of animals, plants, and various organisms and ecosystems. Research in virtually every scientific field may benefit from exploration into the microdose phenomenon.*

The action of the homeopathic medicines ultimately encourages us to acknowledge the intrinsic wisdom of nature through which each organism expresses symptoms in its effort to heal itself. It is indeed a wonder that the bodymind provides clues for determining which medicines can be used in microdose to initiate a healing process. And further, the implications of homeopathic research suggest that we live in a world not of dwindling but increasing resources, if we can only learn to apply them in an optimal manner.

The implications for medicine are stunning. The use of small, specially prepared doses of medicines to stimulate a person's own immune and defense systems can augment, complement, and sometimes replace present medical technologies. The use of microdoses may teach us a new respect for the body and its regenerative capacities. It may help us to realize that we do not have to bombard the body with powerful drugs and risk serious side effects. Small doses, indeed, may sometimes be more powerful and more effective than larger doses.

The implications of homeopathic medicine are truly significant and cry out for more research and replication of past research. Considering how much potential value resides in the field of homeopathy, it would be a crime not to investigate it. Homeopathy is a gold mine waiting for prospectors.

---

*It is important to remember that we are not referring simply to microdoses in general, but to specially prepared microdoses that, when made according to homeopathic procedures, can increase the power of the substance.

Notes

1. Sir William Osler, "Unity, Peace, and Concord—A Farewell Address to the American Medical Profession in 1905," in *The Collected Writings of Sir William Osler* (Birmingham, Ala.: Classics of Medicine Library, 1985), vol. 1; excerpt reprinted in *Journal of the American Medical Association*, 258 (July 3, 1987): 3.

2. David O'Keeffe and M. F. Khan, "Is Homoeopathy a Placebo Response?" *Lancet*, November 8, 1986, pp. 1106–07.

3. David Taylor Reilly, Morag A. Taylor, Charles McSharry, and Tom Aitchison, "Is Homoeopathy a Placebo Response?" *Lancet*, November 29, 1986, p. 1272.

4. Office of Technology Assessment, *Assessing the Safety and Efficacy of Medical Technology* (Washington, D.C.: U.S. Government Printing Office, September 1978), p. 7.

5. Howard P. Bellows, *The Test Drug Proving of the O. O. & L. Society: A Reproving of Belladonna* (Boston: The American Homoeopathic Ophthalmological, Otological, and Laryngological Society, 1906).

6. J. Paterson, "Report on Mustard Gas Experiments," *Journal of the American Institute of Homeopathy*, 37 (1944): 47–50, 88–92.

7. R. M. M. Owen and G. Ives, "The Mustard Gas Experiments of the British Homeopathic Society: 1941–1942," *Proceedings of the 35th International Homeopathic Congress*, 1982, pp. 258–259.

8. David Taylor Reilly, Morag A. Taylor, Charles McSharry, and Tom Aitchison, "Is Homoeopathy a Placebo Response: Controlled Trial of Homoeopathic Potency, with Pollen in Hayfever as Model," *Lancet*, October 18, 1986, pp. 881–886.

9. R. G. Gibson, S. L. M. Gibson, A. D. MacNeil, et al., "Homoeopathic Therapy in Rheumatoid Arthritis: Evaluation by Double-Blind Controlled Trial," *British Journal of Clinical Pharmacology*, 9 (1980): 453–459.

10. Peter Fisher, "An Experimental Double-Blind Trial Method in Homoeopathy: Use of a Limited Range of Remedies to Treat Fibrositis," *British Journal of Homoeopathy*, 74 (1986): 142–147.

11. Henry Albertini et al., "Homeopathic Treatment of Neuralgia Using Arnica and Hypericum: A Summary of 60 Observations," *Journal of the American Institute of Homeopathy*, 78 (September 1985): 126–128.

12. C. F. Claussen, J. Bergmann, G. Bertora, and E. Claussen, "Homöopathische Kombination bei Vertigo und Nausea," *Arzneim.-*

Forsch/Drug Res., 34 (1984): 1791–98.

13. Pierre Dorfman, Marie Noel Lasserre, and Max Tetau, "Preparation à l'accouchement par homéopathie: Expérimentation en double-insu versus placebo" [Preparation for Birth by Homeopathy: Experimentation by Double-blind Versus Placebo], *Cahiers de Biotherapie*, 94 (April 1987): 77–81.

14. M. Shipley, H. Berry, Gill Broster, et al., "Controlled Trial of Homeopathic Treatment of Osteoarthritis," *Lancet*, January 15, 1983, pp. 97–98.

15. C. Oliver Kennedy, "Homoeopathy," *Lancet*, February 26, 1983, p. 482.

16. V. Baumans, C. J. Bol, W. M. T. oude Luttikhuis, and A. C. Beynen, "Does Chelidonium 3x Lower Serum Cholesterol?" *British Homoeopathic Journal*, 76 (January 1987): 14–15.

17. J. C. Cazin et al., "A Study of the Effect of Decimal and Centesimal Dilution of Arsenic on Retention and Mobilization of Arsenic in the Rat," *Human Toxicology*, July 1987.

18. Christopher Day, "Control of Stillbirths in Pigs Using Homoeopathy," *Veterinary Record*, 114 (March 3, 1984): 216; reprinted in *Journal of the American Institute of Homeopathy*, 779 (December 1986): 146–147.

19. Christopher Day, "Clinical Trials in Bovine Mastitis: Use of Nosodes for Prevention," *British Homoeopathic Journal*, 75 (January 1986): 11–15.

20. H. Choudhury, "Cure of Cancer in Experimental Mice with Certain Biochemic Salts," *British Homoeopathic Journal*, 69 (1980): 168–170.

21. G. R. Keysall, K. L. Williamson, and B. D. Tolman, "The Testing of Some Homoeopathic Preparations in Rodents," *Proceedings of the 40th International Homeopathic Congress* (Lyon, France, 1985), pp. 228–231.

22. Adam Sacks, "Nuclear Magnetic Resonance Spectroscopy of Homeopathic Remedies," *Journal of Holistic Medicine*, 5 (Fall–Winter 1983): 172–175; R. B. Smith and G. W. Boericke, "Changes Caused by Succussion on N.M.R. Patterns and Bioassay of Bradykinin Triacetate (BKTA) Succussions and Dilution," *Journal of the American Institute of Homeopathy*, 61 (November–December 1968): 197–212.

23. Jean Boiron, Jacky Abecassis, and Philippe Belon, "The Effects of Hahnemannian Potencies of 7c Histaminum and 7c Apis Mellifica upon Basophil Degranulation in Allergic Patients," *Aspects of Research in Homeopathy* (Lyon: Boiron, 1983), pp. 61–66.

24. J. Sainte Laudy, D. Haynes, and G. Gerswin, "Inhibition of Whole Blood Dilutions on Basophil Degranulation," *International Journal of Immunotherapy*, 2 (1986): 247–250.

25. Elizabeth Davenas, Bernard Poitevin, and Jacques Benveniste, "Effect on Mouse Peritoneal Macrophages of Orally Administered Very High Dilutions of Silica," *European Journal of Pharmacology*, 135 (April 1987): 313–319.

26. L. M. Singh and G. Gupta, "Antiviral Efficacy of Homeopathic Drugs Against Animal Viruses," *British Homoeopathic Journal*, 74 (July 1985): 168–174.

27. W. E. Boyd, "The Action of Microdoses of Mercuric Chloride on Diastase," *British Homoeopathic Journal*, 31 (1941): 1–28; 32 (1942): 106–111.

28. David Mock, "What's Going On Here, Anyway?—A Review of Boyd's 'Biochemical and Biological Evidence of the Activity of High Potencies,'" *Journal of the American Institute of Homeopathy*, 62 (1969): 197.

29. R. L. Jones and M. D. Jenkins, "Comparison of Wheat and Yeast as In Vitro Models for Investigating Homoeopathic Medicines," *British Homoeopathic Journal*, 72 (1983): 143–147.

30. William Steffan, "Growth of Yeast Cultures as In Vitro Model for Investigating Homoeopathic Medicines," *British Homoeopathic Journal*, 73 (October 1984): 198–210.

31. R. D. Baker and C. W. Smith, "Comment on the Paper 'Growth of Yeast Cultures as In Vitro Model for Investigating Homoeopathic Medicines,'" *British Homoeopathic Journal*, 74 (April 1985): 93–95.

32. Jessica Chou, "A Biological Investigation of Succussed Serial Microdilutions," *Journal of the American Institute of Homeopathy*, 79 (September 1986): 100–105.

33. A. R. D. Stebbing, "Hormesis: The Stimulation of Growth by Low Levels of Inhibitors," *The Science of the Total Environment*, 22 (1982): 213–234.

Additional References

For further information on homeopathic research, the following references will be of special aid:

Coulter, Harris L. *Homoeopathic Science and Modern Medicine: The Physics of Healing with Microdoses*. Berkeley: North Atlantic Books, 1981.

Resch, Gerhard, and Viktor Gutmann. *Scientific Foundations of Homoeopathy*. Munich: Bartel and Bartel, 1987.

Scofield, A. M. "Experimental Research in Homoeopathy: A Critical Review." *British Homoeopathic Journal*, 73 (July–October 1984): 161–180, 211–226.

Ullman, Dana, ed. *Monograph on Homeopathic Research*, vols. 1 and 2. Berkeley: Homeopathic Educational Services, 1981, 1986.

Also see the list of homeopathic journals in "Homeopathic Organizations" in Part III, below.

All the above-listed books are available from Homeopathic Educational Services, 2124 Kittredge St., Berkeley, CA 94704.

If you wish to support future scientific investigation of homeopathic medicine, and if you would like updating of information on homeopathic research, contact:

Foundation for Homeopathic Education and Research
5916 Chabot Crest
Oakland, CA 94618

II

The Scope of Homeopathic Practice

Each chapter in the second part of this book discusses the applicability of the medicines to various common and future health problems. These chapters will provide some valuable self-care information, but they are not intended to provide comprehensive medical information. It is recommended that those people interested in learning how to treat acute health problems with homeopathy obtain one or more homeopathic guidebooks. (See "Homeopathic Resources" in Part III.)

4

Pregnancy and Labor: Getting Off to a Good Start

Why is it that so many physicians seem to think that birth is a surgical solution to a nine-month disease? Although good medical care is so important for the health of the mother and infant in high-risk situations, physicians intervene too often in the birthing process, turning normal deliveries into medical emergencies.

The American College of Obstetrics and Gynecology (ACOG) commonly asserts that its members deserve credit for the decline in infant and maternal death rates during the past century. ACOG does not, however, readily acknowledge that most of the countries with the lowest infant mortality rates have the largest numbers of midwives, who provide home births and rarely utilize technological interventions. Despite spending more money per person on health care than any other country, the United States ranks 18th in infant mortality, according to 1984 statistics.[1] It is startling to learn that not only are all the Scandinavian countries ahead of the United States in having lower infant mortality rates, but so are Ireland, Spain, and East Germany.

Despite the various shortcomings of modern obstetrical care, the present regimen is an improvement over the way physicians delivered babies in the 1800s. In the 1870s, women were commonly given regular doses of quinine before birth to prevent fever, plus a powerful cathartic to "cleanse their body," then ergot to induce labor, and morphine to lessen any after pains.[2] The use of these powerful drugs increased, rather than lowered, instances of infant and maternal mortality during childbirth.

With the fear of germs so prominent at the turn of the century, hospitals did all they could to eradicate infectious organisms. Nurses washed women's heads with kerosene, ether, and ammonia. They sometimes shaved pubic hair because they thought that it harbored germs. And they performed enemas on women in labor every twelve hours and gave continual douches of saline solutions to which whisky and bichloride of mercury were added.[3]

The increased effort to protect the mother and infant led to interventions and manipulations of the birthing process that made giving birth both traumatic and dangerous. Describing the 19th-century obstetrician, historians Richard and Dorothy Wertz have also unfortunately characterized the 20th-century obstetrician:

> Doctors were on the lookout for trouble in birth. That seemed to them to be their primary purpose. They found a lot of trouble—so much, in fact, that they came to think that every birth was a potential disaster and that it was best to prepare each woman for the worst eventualities. In line with that perception, doctors increased their control over the patients during labor and delivery, rendering them more powerless to experience or participate in birth. Women acceded to the doctors' increasing control because they also believed that their methods would make birth safer.[4]

The underlying assumption of obstetricians has tended to be that women need technological interventions in order to have a healthy and safe pregnancy and birth. Although some medical interventions are certainly of great value, there is a consensus today that birth has become overmedicalized. Some of this overmedicalization is the result of doctors doing all they can to prevent malpractice suits, and some of it is the result of doctors assuming that more medical interventions improve the chances of having a healthy mother and infant.*

---

*It is rare for physicians to be sued for overutilizing medical interventions, but it is common for suits to arise after a doctor waits before intervention. Dr. David Rubsamen, a physician, attorney, and insurance company consultant, notes: "It's very uncommon for an obstetrician to be

There is now increasing concern about the use of any drugs during pregnancy, since the fetus inevitably receives doses of these drugs, which can disturb its development. Research has shown that drugs during labor and delivery can have short- as well as long-term effects on infants.[5] Even the American Academy of Pediatrics Committee on Drugs has recommended that doctors should "use the smallest possible amount of medications when it is needed, and [should] discuss the benefits and side effects with the mother preferably in advance of the birth."[6]

Obstetricians have contended that the various interventions are necessary for a safe birth. No one can doubt that certain medical interventions can reduce complications and be lifesaving at times. Problems result, however, when conventional drugs and modern technology are utilized in normal or relatively normal childbirths. Obstetricians have ignored the fact that those countries that have utilized the *least* medical interventions during birth have tended to have the best childbirth statistics. Whereas 85 percent of women having hospital delivery in the United States have had an episiotomy, only 8 percent of Dutch women and only 3 percent of Swedish women receive them.[7] Whereas 25–33 percent of women in the United States are aided in birth by a forceps delivery, only about 5 percent of European women receive this treatment.[8] And whereas over 20 percent of American women who have hospital births have a caesarean section, the World Health Organization has conservatively estimated that "there is no justification for any region [of the world] to have a rate higher than 10–15 percent."[9]

Of particular concern to us is that it has been determined that one intervention leads to another, each one increasing health risks to the mother and infant. Drug use during pregnancy causes potential health problems for the fetus and increases the chances of fetal distress syndrome, which may require caesarean section. Amniotomy (the deliberate breaking of the bag of waters surrounding

---

sued because he did an unnecessary Caesarean section. But cases where the charge is that you waited 45 minutes too long are very common." (Fran Smith, "The Losing Battle to Reduce Caesareans," *San Jose Mercury News*, February 17, 1985, p. 1A.)

the baby) helps to induce labor, but as a result the fetus loses the cushion of even pressure that protects it during contractions and lessens compression against the head.

The lithotomy position, in which a woman lies on her back with her feet spread in stirrups is generally convenient for the doctor but is an uncomfortable and inefficient position for women during delivery.* The lithotomy position leads to slower progress of labor, increases chances of the doctor recommending methods to induce and augment labor, often leads to the use of forceps and episiotomy for delivery, and raises blood pressure, which may decrease the amount of oxygen to the fetus, leading to the greater need for caesarean section.

The administration of analgesia and anesthesia to diminish pain during labor decreases the strength and frequency of contractions, usually requiring the use of drugs to augment labor and forceps to aid delivery. These drugs may also lower the mother's blood pressure, which can threaten the life of the fetus. The drugs also prevent the woman from actually feeling how hard she is pushing the baby against her perineum, which may lead to stretching or tearing it. Physicians then must reduce this latter risk with further intervention by doing an episiotomy.

Doing an episiotomy requires local anesthesia, which has the above-mentioned risks associated with it. An episiotomy enables the physician to use forceps to speed up delivery, though there are additional risks to the baby from its application, including hemorrhage within the head and damage to the nerves of the face and arms. There is also an increased threat of severe lacerations of the mother's perineum when forceps and episiotomies are used.

All the above-mentioned interventions increase the chances of needing a caesarean section. The *Canadian Medical Association Journal* has estimated that there are twenty-six times more maternal deaths from caesarean section than from normal delivery.[10] Even when women who had been diagnosed with serious preexisting disease were not counted, the death rate for women

---

*One survey noted that 95 percent of women prefer an upright position during labor and delivery. (Diana Korte and Roberta Scaer, *A Good Birth, A Safe Birth* [New York: Bantam, 1984].)

undergoing a caesarean was still ten times greater.

Since a caesarean section is major surgery that may require a general anesthesia, the mother is unable to breast-feed her infant immediately after birth. And because the mother usually needs to take further medications after this operation, she ultimately is also feeding these drugs to her infant through her breast milk.

Women who are prescribed medications during or after labor, or at any time when they are breast-feeding, are also providing trace amounts of these drugs in their milk. Even though only relatively small amounts of these drugs appear in the milk, the young infant's liver, kidneys, immune system, and general defenses have not matured enough to metabolize and detoxify these drugs effectively. The results may be minor, but in some cases they can be significant.

Drug use during pregnancy can have even more traumatic effects on the new life that is developing in the woman's body.* Thalidomide, an infamous drug that was prescribed to pregnant women in the 1960s and that caused serious birth defects, forced the Food and Drug Administration to require more adequate testing of drugs prior to their availability on the open market. Still, many commonly used drugs can have damaging effects on the fetus, especially when incompatible drugs are utilized together. One expert has estimated that the average pregnant woman in 1980 received four different prescriptions.[11] It is thus no wonder that even conservative statistics now reveal that 12 percent of babies born in the United States have a serious, often incurable mental or physical health disorder.[12]

There is finally a consensus today that drug use during pregnancy, labor, and lactation should be kept to a minimum. However, most physicians in the United States are not aware of specific alternatives to their conventional drugs and thus often have to rely upon them as the primary course of treatment for sick, pregnant, or lactating women. It is a sad fact that American physicians do not know much about homeopathy, and therefore they do not

---

*Drug use during pregnancy is one significant reason for many birth defects, though genetic disposition and exposure to various toxic substances and radiation will also influence the amount of birth defects.

know that homeopathic medicines can be instrumental in diminishing various symptoms of pregnancy, reducing risks of problems in labor, and healing pains, discomforts, or diseases of women who are breast-feeding. Since homeopathic medicines are generally safe, they can provide much benefit and little harm. A growing number of American physicians are finally learning about and using homeopathic medicines. Our children will thank us for this.

Homeopathic Medicines in Pregnancy

The relative safety of homeopathic medicines makes them invaluable during pregnancy, labor, and the postpartum period. "There's nothing safer," says Ananda Zaren, a nurse, midwife, and homeopath in Santa Barbara, California, who has used homeopathic medicines in hundreds of births. Besides being safe, the medicines are quite effective in treating various common problems of pregnancy. Zaren adds: "The medicines help strengthen the woman physically and psychologically."*

Homeopaths have been known to joke that pregnancy is an excellent time to receive homeopathic care, since two people (the mother and the fetus) get a remedy for the price of one. The medicines not only improve the health of the mother but also benefit the fetus. Although no formal statistical analysis has yet been carried out, homeopaths have commonly observed that the children born from women who have received homeopathic care during pregnancy seem healthier than others. Homeopaths make this conjecture by comparing the children of women from previous pregnancies without homeopathic medicines with the offspring of later pregnancies in which the mothers have received the medicines.

It is generally known that the health of the woman greatly affects the health of the fetus. Since pregnancy can be particularly stressful to a woman's body, women often experience exacerbations of previous health problems or various new symptoms. Some of these common symptoms and conditions are nausea, abdominal gas, vaginal infections, bladder infections, herpes, insomnia, ane-

---

*Direct quotes in this and other chapters that do not include a reference derive from personal communications with the author.

mia, backaches, breast swelling and swelling in general, constipation, hemorrhoids, leg cramps, skin eruptions, and varicose veins.

Some of these symptoms and conditions are minor and do not require any treatment with conventional or homeopathic medicines. They can be alleviated with appropriate dietary and lifestyle changes. However, other conditions can be irritating enough to require some kind of treatment. Since pregnant women should be very careful in taking any conventional drugs, it is reasonable and prudent to first consider trying homeopathic medicines for many nonemergency medical conditions.

It is generally recommended that pregnant women receive professional homeopathic care rather than treat themselves. Since their health directly affects the well-being of two people, the pregnant woman deserves the best treatment possible, and an experienced practitioner is better able to provide this care. However, if homeopathic care is not available, individuals can learn to self-prescribe. Unfortunately, there are not many good books on homeopathic medicines for obstetrical problems, and none of the books in English are up-to-date texts. There are some modern texts on homeopathic obstetrics in German and French. (See "Homeopathic Resources" in Part III for information about homeopathic books in English.)

Some women, of course, will be more difficult to treat than others. This book is not intended to get into the technical details of what homeopaths do in such cases. However, it is worthwhile to know that homeopaths differentiate between acute symptoms and chronic symptoms. Acute symptoms represent self-protective efforts of the organism to deal with some type of recent stress or infection. Chronic symptoms, in contrast, represent recurrent, unsuccessful efforts of the organism to reestablish health. Such symptoms may persist because the person is constitutionally weakened from genetic, lifestyle, or environmental factors and/or because the person is continually stressed or frequently reinfected. (This is discussed in more detail in Chapter 9 on "Chronic Diseases.") Sometimes what seems to be an acute symptom is actually the result of an underlying chronic condition. Instead of prescribing a medicine primarily for the most prominent symptom, the homeopath may prescribe a "constitutional" medicine that is individualized to the totality of a woman's symptoms in the light of her present state as well as her family's health history. (See the "Homeopathic Typologies" section in Chapter 1 for more information on what is meant by "constitutional medicine" and "constitutional treatment.")

It is important to bear in mind the distinction between prescriptions for acute and prescriptions for chronic conditions because I will shortly be discussing the individuation of homeopathic medicines for common problems of pregnancy, labor, and the postpartum period. Although several frequently prescribed medicines will be listed for various conditions, homeopaths may prescribe a fundamental or constitutional medicine rather than an acute medicine. It is not appropriate to list all possible constitutional medicines here, both because there are so many of them and because constitutional care should be provided by trained homeopaths.

Homeopaths find that the women who receive constitutional homeopathic treatment prior to becoming pregnant rarely seem to get morning sickness during pregnancy. For those who do get it, there are various homeopathic medicines that are often effective in diminishing the nausea, vomiting, and indigestion common to morning sickness. *Sepia* (cuttlefish), *Nux vomica* (poison nut), *Colchicum* (meadow saffron), *Silica* (silica), *Ipecacuaha* (Ipecac), *Pulsatilla* (windflower), and *Symphoricarpus racemosa* (snowberry) are only a few of the more commonly indicated medicines for morning sickness. All these medicines are known to cause nausea and vomiting when given in overdose and will aid in its cure when given in the microdoses homeopaths use.

To get a sense of the individualization process used in homeopathic medicine, it is worthwhile to differentiate those symptoms that indicate which medicine should be prescribed. Women who need *Sepia, Colchicum, Ipecac,* or *Symphoricarpus* are so nauseous that they cannot even stand the smell of food, though women who need *Sepia* may sometimes feel better after eating. Women who have nausea constantly, not just in the morning, may need *Ipecac, Nux Vomica, Silicea,* or *Symphoricarpus*. Nausea that is ameliorated by lying down indicates *Nux Vomica, Silicea,* or *Symphoricarpus*, while nausea that is aggravated by motion suggests *Ipecac, Sepia,* or *Symphoricarpus. Nux Vomica* is indicated for a type of woman who is highly irritable and who will have symptoms of nausea, vomiting, and constipation worsened in the morning. She will also have a constant pain and pressure in the pit of the stomach and may desire alcohol. *Pulsatilla* is for an emotional woman who is weepy, moody, and indecisive and who has frequent burping of sour, rancid, hot food. She will have nightly diarrhea that tends to change frequently in its color and shape. *Sepia* is given to a woman who has deep feelings of dissatisfaction or indifference. She will have a sense of emptiness at the pit of her stomach, constipation, a bitter or saltish taste in her mouth, and if she is hungry at all, she will desire sour foods. There is general agreement among homeopaths that *Sepia* is the most common medicine prescribed for morning sickness. (More detail about each of these medicines is found in homeopathic texts called *materia medicas*. (See "How to Learn More About Homeopathy" in Part III.)

John Renner, M.D., a homeopath who practiced for over fifty years and who participated in thousands of births, found the best success in giving *Aconite 3x* (monkshood) and *Bryonia 3x* (wild hops) together every thirty minutes. If the woman's symptoms are not noticeably improved within six hours, another remedy should be considered.

It should be candidly noted that some homeopaths find that they successfully cure morning sickness, whereas others find that it is difficult to cure. Homeopath and midwife Ananda Zaren advises: "Sometimes you have to give the woman her constitutional medicine, and at other times the indicated acute medicine is necessary. Although morning sickness is sometimes difficult to treat, homeopathy and sound nutritional advice can provide a safe and sometimes effective treatment for this irritating problem." Morning sickness is not considered a dangerous condition, but since it discourages proper and adequate nutrition, it does present certain risks for the fetus.

Since a homeopathic medicine is prescribed on the basis of the totality of the symptoms the person is experiencing, it is common for women to experience not only relief of their morning sickness from their homeopathic medicine but also a noticeable lessening of various other symptoms. It is, in fact, quite uncommon to see a lasting improvement in nausea without a concurrent general improvement in health. Although no homeopathic research has yet proven that the medicines are beneficial to the mother with morning sickness or to the fetus, clinical experience shows that the medicines have promise for the mother, and the consequential benefits to the fetus are inevitable.

Homeopathic medicines are a literal godsend for many pregnant women who wish to avoid conventional drugs during this special time in their life. Homeopathic medicines are invaluable in treating various irritating symptoms of pregnancy, including vaginal infections, bladder infections, herpes, insomnia, constipation, hemorrhoids, leg cramps, muscle aches, and skin eruptions. Jacques Imberechts, M.D., a respected Belgian homeopath, notes: "The homeopathic medicines are very effective in healing so many symptoms and syndromes of pregnancy that I have found that my patients rarely request or need anything other than homeopathic treatment." Dr. Imberechts admits that he has had difficulty in treating women who develop varicose veins during pregnancy, though he personally feels that constitutional care before and during pregnancy can possibly prevent this condition. Richard Moskowitz, M.D., a Boston homeopath, has found the best results with *Pulsatilla* and *Hamamelis* (witch hazel) in treating varicose veins. Marcel Simons, M.D., a Belgian obstetrician and homeopath, has also observed good results with these medicines as well as with *Vipera* (the German viper).

Homeopathic Medicines During Labor

Besides using homeopathic medicines to diminish the pain and discomfort of pregnancy, the medicines can also be used to prepare the women for the process of labor. Homeopaths have often cited numerous instances in which the properly indicated medicine has helped to turn a breech baby. *Pulsatilla* is a common medicine for this, though the best medicine is generally the one indicated based on the uniqueness of each woman's symptoms. Ananda Zaren notes that the medicines *can* turn a breech baby late in pregnancy, though they seem to work faster in turning breech babies that occur early in pregnancy. Zaren asserts that a footling breech, a rare position during labor in which one foot or both come down first, represents a structural problem for the woman and cannot be treated effectively with homeopathic medicines.

By turning breech presentations, homeopathic medicines can change a higher-risk pregnancy into a normal one. Because the medicines offer so much potential for benefit during pregnancy and little potential for side effects, homeopathic medicines will inevitably play an increasingly important role in childbirth in the near future and in the 21st century.

John George, M.D., a Seattle obstetrician and gynecologist, utilizes homeopathic medicines in his practice and has found that "in many ways the medicines facilitate the childbirth process for the woman and the physician. The medicines make it all go a lot more smoothly." Specifically, Dr. George notes: "The correctly prescribed homeopathic remedy given in preparation and anticipation of labor is observed to prepare the cervix for labor by facilitating and softening, thinning out, and dilating the cervix prior to the onset of real labor. The second observation is that the labor pattern of contractions tends to be more orderly and efficient in progressing the birth. Thirdly, the amount of pain experienced during labor is markedly reduced, greatly lessening the need for analgesics and anesthesia."

Ananda Zaren notes that constitutional medicines are rarely indicated during labor, since the process of childbirth creates stresses that require the use of medicine for acute symptoms. Zaren has found that the microdoses prevent problems during delivery, decrease delivery time, and increase the woman's pain threshold so that she can deal with the pain of childbirth more easily.

Homeopaths, like good conventional physicians, prefer not to prescribe any medicines if it seems that the labor is normal and healthy. The homeopath, however, has at his or her disposal several medicines that can help the process if there are any complications. *Caulophyllum* (blue cohosh), for example, is a medicine par excellence in strengthening uterine muscles, which can help the process of labor. It is not the only medicine prescribed for this condition, but it is the most commonly given remedy. Generally, the 3rd, 6th, 12th, 30th, or 200th potency is given if the woman's labor is progressing slowly and if the woman has an undilated cervix that may be spasmodically rigid and with feeble contractions.

Caulophyllum is also indicated if the contractions are irregular or if there is atony (weakness) of the uterus during labor. Dr. Jacques Imberechts half-jokingly says: "When it seems like labor is beginning, you should call the taxi and then take *Caulophyllum*. If you take the medicine before you call the taxi, you're likely to have that baby in the taxi."

French researchers recently completed a double-blind trial using *Caulophyllum* and four other homeopathic medicines to treat pregnant women.* The study found that the homeopathic medicine significantly reduced childbirth time and decreased abnormal labor. Ninety-three women were involved in the experiment; forty were given a placebo and fifty-three were given a 5c combination medicine. The researchers found that women given the homeopathic medicine were in labor for an average of 5.1 hours, while those given a placebo were in labor for an average of 8.5 hours. Only 11.3 percent of the women given the homeopathic medicine had an abnormal labor, while 40 percent of those given a placebo had an abnormal labor.[13]

In addition to research on humans, studies on animals confirm the value of *Caulophyllum* in labor. In a British study of over 200 births, it was shown to reduce significantly the numbers of stillbirths in a herd of pigs with a high stillbirth rate.[14]

Respected British homeopath Douglas Borland recommended taking *Caulophyllum 12* or *30* daily during the last two or three weeks of pregnancy as a way to strengthen and prepare the woman for childbirth.[15] Some other homeopaths feel that one should never routinely give *Caulophyllum*, but that each woman must be individually treated.

Belladonna (deadly nightshade) and *Cimicifuga* (black snakeroot) are two other commonly indicated medicines for helping the process of labor. *Belladonna* is indicated when the woman experiences some of the characteristic symptoms of this medicine, which include an extreme nervousness and agitation, deliriousness, general flushing of the face and mucous membranes, and hot skin.

---

*Other remedies included in this medicine were *Actea dracemosa* (cimicifuga or black snakeroot), *Arnica* (mountain daisy), *Pulsatilla* (windflower), and *Gelsemium* (yellow jasmine).

Women who need *Cimicifuga* tend to be somewhat hysterical, frequently sighing, experiencing spasmodic pains that seem to fly in various directions, and being intolerant of the pain. A characteristic symptom of those who need *Cimicifuga* is pessimism about the labor, with the woman proclaiming such things as "I can't do it" or "this is driving me crazy; I can't take it anymore."

There are several other homeopathic medicines that should be considered, depending on the woman's individual symptoms. Prescribing homeopathic medicines during labor provides yet another opportunity for safe alternatives to conventional medications.

The Homeopathic Treatment of Mother and Infant

The process of labor can be exhausting. If the woman is worn out or if she has muscle aches from the physical exertion, *Arnica* (mountain daisy) is indicated. *Arnica* is discussed in greater detail in Chapter 10 on "Sports Medicine," for it is known as a superb medicine for aches and pains of overexertion and for shock and trauma of injury. Though childbirth is not exactly an "injury," it does put a woman's body through a certain amount of shock and trauma. *Arnica* is also valuable after delivery for the mother and the infant, since it is so effective in helping both of them to recoup from the childbirth process. (Homeopathic medicines are safe for infants, though it is recommended that one give them only small homeopathic pellets—or crush the larger pellets into small pieces—so that infants do not choke on them. One can also place the pellets in water and then feed an infant with a clean teaspoon or dropper.)

Homeopathic medicines can also be used to help the mother recuperate from the drama and trauma of labor that requires medical intervention. If an episiotomy or a caesarean is performed, homeopaths commonly give the woman *Staphysagria* (stavesacre), a major medicine that homeopaths give after surgery. Homeopaths have observed that women who take *Staphysagria* do not seem to request painkillers after labor as often as other women do.

Dr. John George has found good results with *Sulphur* after a long or difficult labor. He has also noted that "the stretching and tearing of the tissues around the bladder, perineal area, and vulva shower bacteria into the surrounding tissues and into the bloodstream, which can cause a bladder infection or other complications, all of which *Sulphur* seems to prevent effectively."

If the mother has torn her perineum during delivery, British homeopath Robert Davidson recommends *Bellis perrenis 200c* (daisy). He has found that it works well in these internal injuries. *Calendula tincture* is also of value in speeding the healing process. This salve is generally applied with a wet sponge.

If the infant is asphyxiated, conventional medical measures are necessary, though homeopathic medicine can still increase the chances of survival. *Antimonium tart* (tartar emetic) is one of the most common medicines that homeopaths give to asphyxiated babies. A baby may seem dead, though more often he will have a rattling in his throat and breathing difficulties due to some phlegm blocking his respiration. *Antimonium tart* seems to help the baby remove the phlegm immediately. Generally, if *Antimonium tart* does not work, *Carbo veg* (vegetable charcoal) or *Camphor* (camphor) may be needed. Those babies who require *Carbo veg* tend to be cold and blue. Those babies who need *Camphor* usually have a high fever, a deep redness over the entire abdomen and thighs, and tetanic spasms. *Opium* (opium) is another homeopathic medicine that can be indicated if the baby is unconscious and rigid throughout the whole body. It also tends to be needed if the mother experiences a profound fear either during her pregnancy or during labor. *Laurocerasus* (cherry laurel) is valuable if the baby has a facial twitch when gasping for air. *Arnica* (mountain daisy) is indicated after a baby has experienced a traumatic delivery evidenced by a hematoma (blood and swelling) on the skull. *Arnica*, like *Opium*, is also indicated when the baby has a bodily stiffness, but *Arnica* is preferred if the baby also has a hot face, cold body, jerking respiration, and tremor of the limbs.

Homeopaths have found that the correctly prescribed medicine tends to work immediately, which, considering the circumstances, is necessary for the baby's survival. The prescription of any of these medicines should not delay the other heroic medical measures necessary to aid the baby's chances of survival.

Homeopaths also report success in treating neonatal jaundice.

They find that the correct medicine can resolve this condition in one to three days. Conventional treatment usually requires hospitalization, in which the baby is put in an incubator and exposed to special fluorescent lights that break down bilirubin and encourage healthy liver function. It usually takes three days to two weeks to resolve this condition. Of particular significance, the incubation of the baby separates him or her from the mother, making breast-feeding difficult or impossible. This separation also significantly reduces the amount of skin-to-skin contact, which is so valuable physiologically and psychologically to both the infant and the mother.

Alphonse Teste, M.D., a famous 19th-century French homeopath, asserted, with reference to neonatal jaundice, that *Aconite* (monkshood) "will often suffice to cure the disease."[16] If improvement is not observed within twenty-four hours, *Nux vomica* (poison nut), *Chelidonium* (celandine), *Lycopodium* (club moss), *Chionanthus* (fringe-tree), *Bovista* (puffball), or *Natrum sulph* (sulphate of sodium) should all be considered.

Besides aiding women in pregnancy and labor, homeopathic medicines can also be helpful to a mother who develops problems that make breast-feeding difficult. Breast-feeding, of course, plays a very important role in providing the newborn baby with important antibodies, enzymes, and other essential nutrients that help the baby adapt to and thrive in his or her new surroundings. Women with mastitis (inflammation of the breast) need to be treated as soon as possible so that they can continue breast-feeding. Dr. Robert Mendelsohn, a well-known pediatrician and author, feels that breast-feeding is so important that physicians and others should do all they can to encourage it. Dr. Mendelsohn counters those people who say that it is disgusting to breast-feed in public by claiming that it is more disgusting to bottle-feed in public.

Mastitis, incidentally, is one of the most common breast problems after childbirth. Conventional treatment for this condition is simply to administer antibiotics. Although these drugs work reasonably well, it certainly would be worthwhile to try an alternative treatment that is safe and effective, since the baby will end up receiving trace amounts of the antibiotics through the breast milk. *Belladonna, Bryonia, Phytolacca* (pokeroot), and *Lac cani-*

num (dog's milk) are the most commonly effective medicines for mastitis. *Belladonna* and *Bryonia* are most often given at the first stages of mastitis. *Belladonna* is indicated when the woman has red, hot, and swollen breasts, which, like *Lac caninum*, are very sensitive to motion or jarring. Women who need *Belladonna* will have a high fever, congestion in the head, throbbing headache, and flushed face. *Bryonia* should be prescribed when the breasts have a stony hardness in them. The breasts will be hot and painful, but not very red. There may be a sharp, stitching pain that is made worse by motion, especially by raising the arm. The woman will have dry lips, thirst, and constipation.

Women who need *Phytolacca* have stony-hard and very painful breasts that are discharging pus. There may be an excessive flow of milk, though the nipples are so sensitive that nursing produces intense suffering that radiates all over the body. Women who need *Lac caninum* have sore and tender breasts that are particularly sensitive to motion or even the slightest jar. They experience pain while walking or sometimes by simple inspiration, though this pain diminishes if the woman supports her breasts when moving in any way.

There are numerous problems of pregnancy, labor, and the postpartum period that have not been discussed in this chapter. Since homeopathic medicines strengthen the individual's overall health, they can be applied in general to treat a wide variety of acute or chronic obstetrical conditions. The history and present worldwide use of these medicines provide some evidence of their value. Homeopathic medicines will probably not only be invaluable to our children in the 21st century, but to their children as well.

Notes

1. 1986 World Population Data Sheet, Population Reference Bureau (777 14th St., NW, Washington, D.C. 20005).

2. Richard W. Wertz and Dorothy C. Wertz, *Lying-In: A History of Childbirth in America* (New York: Schocken, 1979), p. 137.

3. Ibid., p. 138.

4. Ibid., p. 136.

5. Diana Korte and Roberta Scaer, *A Good Birth, A Safe Birth* (New York: Bantam, 1984), pp. 113–137.

6. Ibid., pp. 129–130.

7. Ibid., pp. 132–133.

8. Ibid., p. 134.

9. World Health Organization, "Appropriate Technology for Birth," *Lancet*, 8452 (August 24, 1985): 436.

10. Quoted in Herbert H. Keyser, *Women Under the Knife* (New York: Warner, 1984), p. 72.

11. Robert Mendelsohn, *Male Practice: How Doctors Manipulate Women* (Chicago: Contemporary Books, 1982).

12. Mark Dowie, "Terata," *Mother Jones*, January 1985, pp. 14–21.

13. Pierre Dorfman, Marie Noel Lasserre, and Max Tetau, "Preparation à l'accouchement par homéopathie: Expérimentation en double-insu versus placebo" [Preparation for Birth by Homeopathy-Experimentation by Double-blind Versus Placebo], *Cahiers de Biotherapie*, 94 (April 1987): 77–81.

14. C. E. I. Day, "Control of Stillbirths in Pigs Using Homoeopathy," *British Homoeopathic Journal*, 73 (July 1984): 142–143.

15. Douglas M. Borland, *Homoeopathy for Mother and Infant* (New Delhi: B. Jain, n.d.).

16. T. C. Duncan, *Disease of Infants and Children and Their Homoeopathic Treatment* (Chicago: Duncan Brothers, 1880), vol. 2, p. 492.

Additional References

Edwards, Margot, and Mary Waldot. *Reclaiming Birth*. Trumansburg, N.Y.: Crossing Press, 1984.

Fisher, Charles. *A Handbook on the Diseases of Children and Their Homoeopathic Treatment*. Chicago: Medical Century, 1895.

Goer, Henci. "Are Cesareans Saving Babies?: A Review of the Medical Literature." *Childbirth Alternatives Quarterly*, 7 (Summer 1986): 9–11.

Hamlin, Frederick W. *A Manual of Practical Obstetrics*. New York: Boericke and Runyon, 1908.

Hotchner, Tracy. *Pregnancy and Childbirth*. New York: Avon, 1979.

Isaacs, Janet Ashford. "Trends in World Infant Mortality." *Childbirth Alternative Quarterly*, 8 (Fall 1986): 13.

Society of Homeopaths. "Homeopathy in Pregnancy, Childbirth, and Childhood." Proceedings from a Seminar Held in London on November 1, 1980.

Tyler, Margaret. "Mastitis." *Homoeopathy*, 7 (January 1938): 3–8.

Yingling, W. A. *The Accoucheur's Emergency Manual.* New Delhi: B. Jain, n.d.

5

Pediatrics: Don't Drug Our Kids—Give Them Homeopathics

Earlier in this century, meningitis was fatal 95 percent of the time in children who contracted it. Now, because of the use of antibiotics, 95 percent of the children who get it survive. The number of infants dying in the first two years of life has also dramatically declined, once again primarily because of the use of conventional medicine. The significant reduction in the number of children dying from leukemia is another impressive development of modern medicine. Despite these benefits of modern medicine, however, there is general agreement that medical care can and should be better. There is also recognition that modern medicine is not always safe and that, in fact, it sometimes does more harm than good.

Medical Child Abuse

Benjamin Rush, M.D. (1745–1813), considered the "father of American medicine," was such an advocate of bloodletting* that

---

*Bloodletting is the use of a knife (called a lancet) to cut into a vein to release blood. Although this therapy did at least temporarily reduce the redness and swelling of inflammation, it also greatly weakened already sick people. Bloodletting was so respected that a major British medical journal called itself *Lancet*, under which name it is still published today.

he even recommended it for sick newborn infants.[1] Rush asserted that physicians who did not bloodlet their patients were quacks. This barbaric treatment is no longer recommended, though one must wonder if the way we are presently treating children with powerful drugs, often given repeatedly and in combination with other drugs, will be considered barbaric at some time in the future.

Conservative use of conventional drugs with newborns, infants, and children is recommended, since their bodies are still developing, the organs and glands are learning how to function in concert, and the immune and defense reactions are in the process of maturation. It is now (finally!) acknowledged that pregnant women should avoid medications during pregnancy; and yet, once our children are born, we seem to forget that their bodies are still in the process of growth and development, a delicate state that can be significantly affected by many commonly used medications.

It is a little known fact that the vast majority of drugs commonly used for infant and child health problems have not been adequately tested on pediatric populations. Even a report from the American Academy of Pediatrics admitted that "possibly as many as three quarters of the drugs used in hospital pediatric practice are not officially approved for the purpose for which they are commonly employed."[2]

As recently as 1975, 95 percent of physicians gave children one or more prescriptions for the common cold, and about 60 percent of the time one of the drugs was an antibiotic.[3] In 1979, the Food and Drug Administration (FDA) found thirty drugs to be ineffective, more than half of which were often prescribed for children.[4]

In 1975, the American Academy of Pediatrics recommended that tetracycline not be given to children under eight years old because it can retard bone growth, damage the liver, cause various digestive upsets, and even permanently stain the child's teeth. And yet, a study in 1977 showed that 27 percent of 1,947 Tennessee physicians surveyed prescribed tetracycline to children under eight.[5] Although some conventional drugs are, no doubt, more dangerous than others for children, there is little controversy about the fact that we must use drugs with greater caution in the treatment of infants and children than in the treatment of adults.

During pregnancy, the fetus is protected by the mother's antibodies, which regularly are fed through the umbilical cord. After birth, the mother's milk is also filled with important antibodies and nutrients, which are invaluable for helping to build the immune and defense systems of the newborn baby. At the tender age of only two months, the baby begins to experience the six to nine viral infections per year that he (or she) will experience until the end of his childhood. Usually manifesting itself in a common cold, each virus is eventually fought off, and in the process the baby's immune system is exercised and strengthened.

Fever is the way in which the body heats up in an effort to create an internal environment unconducive to viral growth. During this fevered state, the body's white blood cells become more active, and more interferon is produced, which aids in fighting the viral infection.* It is no wonder, then, that aspirin has been found to lead to Reyes Syndrome, a potentially fatal neurological condition, when given to suppress children's fever.

Nasal discharge is further evidence of a child's effort to heal. The discharge is primarily dead viruses, dead bacteria, dead white blood cells, and mucus. The use of nasal sprays, decongestants, and antihistamines inhibits this elimination, which is a natural defense of the body. The suppression of the nasal discharge makes no sense physiologically, which is probably the reason that such treatments usually do not work and often cause various side effects that are generally worse than the simple cold the child initially had.

Children are frequently given cough suppressants, too. Since a cough is a natural defense of the body in its efforts to clear a breathing passageway, it is physiologically counterproductive to routinely give cough suppressants to children. And to make matters worse, many of the most popular cold and cough remedies have 50- to 80-proof alcohol in them. A 1984 report from the American Academy of Pediatrics warned that "even small amounts of alcohol can affect a child's central nervous system, causing decreased reaction time, muscular incoordination, and behavioral

---

*Interferon is a natural protein of the body that inhibits virus multiplication.

changes."[6]

When a person gets something done for him, he does not learn to do it himself. Likewise, on a physiological and immunological level, when drugs are given to treat a symptom or infection, the body does not learn to heal itself as well on its own.

The Homeopathic Alternative to Aspirin in Fevers

Homeopathic medicine offers an alternative to drugs that suppress symptoms. Even a book written in 1858 that was critical of homeopathy admitted that homeopathic medicines were "decided favorites with the children."[7]

Although there are those rare instances when an infant's or child's fever is so high that some type of treatment, even if it be suppressive, is recommended, homeopathic medicines are often effective in rapidly curing such conditions.* *Aconite* (monkshood) and *Belladonna* (deadly nightshade) are two common homeopathic remedies for infant fevers. These herbs are known to be toxic, but in the small doses that homeopaths use, they are valuable and safe therapeutic agents.

Sidney Ringer (1835–1910), the British physiologist who developed "Ringer's Solution" (a commonly used salt solution for intravenous fluids), proclaimed that "no drug is more valuable than *Aconite*" for its ability to control inflammation.[8] Even Joseph Lister (1827–1912), one of England's most respected surgeons, recognized its value. Lister noted that he derived his knowledge of *Aconite* and *Belladonna* from the homeopaths.[9]

The symptoms of children who need *Aconite* or *Belladonna* have similarities, but they have individualizing differences as well. Both symptoms may begin with a sudden onset of fever, and both

---

*For detailed guidelines on when medical care is indicated, see Stephen Cummings and Dana Ullman, *Everybody's Guide to Homeopathic Medicines* (Los Angeles: J. P. Tarcher, 1984); Robert Mendelsohn, *How to Raise a Healthy Child . . . In Spite of Your Doctor* (Chicago: Contemporary Books, 1984); and Robert Pantell, James Fries, and Donald Vickery, *Taking Care of Your Child* (Reading, Mass.: Addison-Wesley, 1977).

may even develop into a very high fever. However, although both medicines are primarily useful during the initial stages of fever, they are not useful for those fevers that are protracted. *Aconite* is commonly given to infants or children who develop their condition after exposure to dry and cold air or wind, especially if they had been perspiring during that exposure. *Aconite* is also for infants or children who, along with the fever, have dry skin, a dry cough, a dry mouth, and sometimes an unquenchable thirst, generally for cold drinks. They are mentally alert, though they are also usually anxious, restless, and fearful. They may toss in their sleep or throw off their covers or clothes.

Infants or children who need *Belladonna* look distinctively different. They have a red, flushed face, intensely hot skin (which may even radiate heat, allowing the parent to feel the heat without touching the child), and glassy eyes with dilated pupils. They are mentally delirious and do not seem to comprehend what is going on around them. Their illness generally makes them lethargic and mentally dull. Rather than the *Aconite* child's restlessness and fear, the *Belladonna* child has restlessness with mental dullness and confusion. If these children have a high fever, they may hit, bite, or tear at things. They may also experience wild dreams or, in severe cases, may say they see monsters and other hallucinations. In certain cases, these children may develop muscle twitchings, which seem to come and go suddenly.

Some of the symptoms of *Belladonna* are also symptoms of meningitis, which many homeopaths feel they frequently avert with the use of homeopathic medicines. If a child is diagnosed as having meningitis, however, homeopaths do not resist using antibiotics, since meningitis is a condition too serious to delay treatment. One of the extra benefits of using homeopathy in infants' or children's fevers is that the medicines generally work extremely rapidly. And if the incorrect medicine is given, no side effects occur.

Convulsions with fever in infants who do not have meningitis are not uncommon. Too often these infants are given powerful anticonvulsive medications. Parents should know that there is no evidence that infants will suffer serious aftereffects from these convulsions. One study of 1,706 children with febrile convulsions

showed that they did not lead to a single death or motor defect.[10]
There is also no convincing evidence that febrile seizures lead to
epilepsy later in life. Severe recurrent seizures, however, can cause
brain damage, and conventional or homeopathic treatment for
them is important. However, treatment for the common febrile
seizures with anticonvulsive medications is inappropriate and
dangerous.

Homeopathic doses of *Belladonna, Chamomilla, Calcarea
carbonica* (calcium carbonate), *Helleborus* (snow-rose), *Opium*
(opium), *Stramonium* (thorn-apple), *Nux vomica* (poison nut), and
Zinc (zinc) are among the safer homeopathic alternatives to conventional anticonvulsive medications. For best results in treating
this condition, it is generally recommended to seek professional
homeopathic care.

The Homeopathic Treatment of Common Infant Health Problems: Teething, Colic, and Eczema

Shakespeare once described infancy as the age of "mewling and
puking in the nurse's arms." Although there are innumerable
theories for why infants vomit or have one condition or another,
the underlying basis of homeopathic thought is that symptoms are
responses of the organism to deal with infections or some type of
internally or externally derived stress. Symptoms, then, represent
the best efforts of the body to try to defend and heal itself.

Besides the inappropriate treatment of infant fevers and colds,
another common, inappropriate treatment that is often administered is for infants' teething problems. A large group of pediatricians were recently surveyed about what they do for teething infants. Virtually all prescribed medications, usually painkillers of
varying strengths, sedatives, and local anesthetics.[11]

It is certainly understandable that parents want to do something to allay their infants' pain during the teething stage. Besides
the tooth pain and drooling that infants suffer, they also often have
fever, bowel problems (usually diarrhea, or constipation alternating with diarrhea), colds, and skin rashes. And it is certainly
understandable that physicians who see the pained infants and

the frightened and concerned parents would want to do something. However, homeopathy offers such an effective alternative to problems associated with teething that physicians and parents will inevitably look to it.

Chamomilla has probably introduced more parents to homeopathy than any other homeopathic medicine. It is not the only medicine that homeopaths prescribe to treat teething, but it is so commonly used that it is generally recommended unless the infant's symptoms clearly indicate the need for a different medicine. The most common symptoms of infants who need *Chamomilla* are inflamed gums, drooling, and a desire to keep fingers in the mouth. Commonly, one cheek is hot and red, while the other is pale. More notable than these physical symptoms are the emotional and behavioral changes. The infants are hyperirritable and may scream and hit. They demand things, but reject them as soon as they are given. During sleep they toss and turn and may cry aloud. The only relief they experience comes when they are being carried about or rocked. This description of *Chamomilla* infants no doubt sounds familiar to many parents.

Other homeopathic medicines given to teething infants are *Calcarea phosphorica* (phosphate of calcium), *Calcarea carbonica* (calcium carbonate), and *Coffea* (coffee).

For numerous infant and childhood conditions, it may often be more appropriate to treat the parent's anxiety than the pediatric complaint. The fever-phobia that parents have and the fear that any symptom requires immediate treatment is a common, though "curable," state of mind. Although there are certainly conditions that require medical attention, the vast majority of infant and childhood symptoms are nothing to worry about. Pediatrician Robert Mendelsohn has noted that 95 percent of pediatric ailments heal themselves and do not require medical care.[12]

One important recommendation for parents who want to try to treat their children is to remember to avoid treatments that suppress symptoms. Treatments that try to counteract the body's natural defensive tendencies are generally suppressive. One example of a common home treatment for infants' colic (or sometimes for children's digestive problems, too) is the use of baking soda. Although baking soda may neutralize the stomach acids, it causes what is called a "rebound effect," in which the body reacts to the baking soda by secreting even more stomach acids.

The homeopathic alternative to treating infants' colic and children's digestive problems is an individually chosen homeopathic medicine. *Chamomilla* is one of the common medicines for colic when the infant has the typically hyperirritable state that is normally associated with this medicine, as described earlier. *Pulsatilla* (windflower) is another common medicine for colic, but the infants for whom it is prescribed are generally very affectionate and desirous of attention and sympathy; although they may be irritable from the pain they experience, they are still basically friendly. Some of the other commonly used homeopathic medicines for colicky infants are *Arsenicum* (arsenic), *Nux vomica* (poison nut), *Bryonia* (wild hops), *Magnesia phosphorica* (phosphate of magnesia), *Colocynthis* (bitter cucumber), *Lycopodium* (club moss), and *Sulphur* (sulphur). There are numerous other homeopathic medicines (too many to list here) that are occasionally given to colicky infants.

Some people theorize that the reason for colic is that the infant is allergic to milk or to some other food. The homeopathic view of food allergies is basically that the food is not "the problem." Rather, it is the individual's underlying state of health. The disease process produces poor assimilation and utilization of the food, which then ultimately creates symptoms. Homeopaths have found that the homeopathic medicines are effective in reestablishing health and thereby reducing food allergies. (See Chapter 8 for more information on the homeopathic approach to treating allergies.)

Eczema is another common infant disease. Conventional medical treatment of this condition is again a sad example of symptom suppression. Homeopaths understand that skin diseases (as distinct from injuries to the skin or symptoms from exposure to irritants) are not simply skin problems but are the result of an underlying internal disorder. Using cortisone or other strong steroidal medicines suppresses the natural defensive effort of the body. Although they are sometimes highly effective in suppressing symptoms, they do not treat the internal disease.

Systemic cortisone taken orally or by injection causes significantly more serious side effects than topical cortisone creams, but even these creams are not harmless. Although few serious symptoms have been attributed to the cortisone creams, it is very difficult to assess their long-term effects.

Parents often note that the eczema returns, sometimes worse than before, when cortisone treatment is stopped. For the "lucky" ones, the eczema may not come back; however, from a homeopathic point of view, this may be either a good or a bad sign. It may mean that the infant has finally "grown out of the condition," or it may mean that the internal condition has been driven deeper into the body, ultimately to manifest itself in a more serious disease. Most commonly, homeopaths see the suppression of skin symptoms later resulting in a lung condition, usually asthma.* Since the skin does much breathing for the body and acts as a "third lung," it is predictable that disease would attack the superficial lung first. Then, as the condition is either ineffectively treated or suppressed, it attacks the two primary sources of life's breath.

Homeopaths understand eczema as an internal disorder, so they need to choose a remedy individually based on a full evaluation of the infant's physical, emotional, and mental characteristics as well as his or her genetic endowment. It is thus recommended that one seek professional homeopathic care rather than attempting homeopathic home care. An infant's body is still in a delicate stage of development and should be treated with the utmost care.

Homeopathic Treatment of Childhood Conditions

Benjamin Spock once said that a child who has never bumped his head is being too closely watched. One of the most common health

---

*Conventional physicians commonly note that eczema and asthma are linked, although they, unlike homeopaths, generally treat them as separate illnesses and prescribe different medications for them. These physicians do not recognize this internalizing of the disease as suppression or as a worsening of the child's illness. Homeopaths assume that whenever treatment simply controls or suppresses symptoms, true cure will remain elusive, and disease is likely to penetrate deeper into the person.

problems of children is accidents. Although homeopathy has developed its reputation by its successful treatment of acute and chronic disease, it is also of great benefit in injuries. *Arnica* (mountain daisy) has introduced countless numbers of parents to homeopathy because of its impressively rapid action in diminishing pain from blows to the head or to the soft tissue. Because of its effects on injuries to soft tissue, it is the most common medicine for injuries that become black and blue. (For more detailed information on injuries, see Chapter 10 on "Sports Medicine.")

Many previously common childhood illnesses (measles, German measles, mumps, whooping cough, diphtheria) are now rare. For some of these conditions this decrease was largely the result of immunizations, and for others it was merely their natural evolution as infectious diseases. Homeopathy offers relatively effective treatment for these conditions, but it is not worthwhile discussing this subject because of the rare appearance of these diseases. Chicken pox, on the other hand, is one of the persisting childhood illnesses for which homeopathy offers treatment. Homeopaths have noted, in particular, that microdoses seem to prevent the complications that occasionally result from chicken pox.

Although there are several medicines that should be considered, the most common chicken pox remedy is *Rhus tox* (poison ivy). *Rhus tox* is effective in treating chicken pox because it causes itching and burning skin symptoms similar to this condition. Other medicines that should be considered are *Pulsatilla* (windflower), *Antimonium tart* (tartar emetic), *Antimonium crudum* (black sulphide of antimony), *Arsenicum* (arsenic), *Belladonna* (deadly nightshade), and *Mercurius* (mercury).

Homeopathy is also effective in treating common infectious diseases of childhood, including ear infections and strep throat. (For a detailed description of this treatment, see Chapter 7 on "Infectious Diseases.")

One of the more common childhood difficulties is what is often called "hyperactivity." It is also sometimes called "attention deficit disorder," "learning disability," or "minimal brain damage." Although it seems that many children are hyperactive, only a relatively small percentage of those seem to be truly ill. Many children simply have boundless energy, get bored easily, and have little interest in learning certain school subjects. Most children eventually outgrow this hyperactive stage without any noticeable problems.

Hyperactivity as an illness does, however, exist. It manifests itself in poor learning, disruptive behavior, and poor relationships with friends, siblings, and other family members. Conventional physicians most often prescribe *Ritalin* (methylphenidate), an amphetamine-like drug. It is indeed ironic that physicians would consider giving an amphetamine-like drug to children who are hyperactive. One would think that this drug would make the children even more hyperactive. But *Ritalin* has a noticeably opposite effect on such children. It calms them down and allows them to play or to sit and learn without behavioral disruption.

Conventional physicians refer to the "paradoxical action" of drugs as the reason that *Ritalin* works. But "paradoxical action" is just another name for the homeopathic "law of similars." The drug does not further relax children who are already calm; it only calms those who are hyperactive. Because *Ritalin* normally *causes* hyperactivity, it can treat it effectively.

Although *Ritalin* is generally effective in temporarily relieving hyperactivity, it is a powerful drug that has side effects. *Ritalin* and other amphetamine drugs used to treat hyperactivity can cause nervousness, insomnia, reduced appetite, weight loss, retarded growth, stomachaches, skin rashes, headaches, and hallucinations. Of particular importance, it is largely unknown what long-term effects these drugs have on the fragile bodies of children.

Hyperactivity in children is another condition that requires professional homeopathic care. Some of the commonly prescribed medicines for this condition are *Argenticum nitricum* (silver nitrate), *Arsenicum* (arsenic), *Phosphorus* (phosphorus), *Hepar sulphur* (Hahnemann's calcium sulphide), *Tuberculinum* (tubercle bacilli), *Sulphur* (sulphur), *Staphysagria* (stavesacre), *Nux vomica* (poison nut), and *Zinc* (zinc).

To give the reader a sense of two of these common types, a comparison of *Argenticum nitricum* and *Arsenicum* will be helpful. It is fitting that silver should be used to treat hyperactivity, since this metal is one of the most highly conductive substances known. Children who need *Argenticum nitricum* can easily, perhaps too easily, transmit energy, like silver itself. They constantly hurry and are ridden with anxiety. They experience great anticipation about performing, whether it be for an examination or a school play. They are unable to fix their attention. They often try to explain themselves and their behavior. They are master rationalizers, though most of their explanations are irrational (some people, however, may call their explanations "creative"). Physically, they may look older than they are. They walk faster than others. They have a great craving for sugar, even though some of their physical or psychological symptoms may appear soon afterwards. They do not need as much clothing as others, are usually aggravated by warmth, and feel better in cool environments. They may experience incoordination or even trembling. They may have much gas and may have stomach pains.

Hyperactive children who need *Arsenicum* have a driving restlessness. They are very anxious, over something specific or just things in general. They have an anticipation that something bad may happen, especially when they are alone. Whenever possible, they avoid being alone and do what they can to be around others. They are very possessive and fastidious. They will not let others play with their toys, and, if necessary, they may play with all their toys at once to thwart other kids from doing so. In general, their desires are greater than their needs, a situation that is expressed in their having constantly changing and expanding desires. They can have a fussy meticulousness that may manifest itself in their being very orderly or in their doing things just "the right way."

In part as a result of their hyperactivity, children who need *Arsenicum* undergo stages of exhaustion and weakness. They are hypersensitive to odors, touch, and noise, and may have physical or psychological reactions to milk, wheat, sugar, or ice cream. They easily become chilly, and exposure to cold may bring on a cold, cough, or headache. They become better from most forms of heat. They often have a great thirst, but prefer to drink only sips at a time. They sometimes get exacerbations of physical symptoms at midnight, often causing them difficulty staying asleep.

The distinct symptoms of *Argenticum nitricum* and *Arsenicum* clearly show how different children experience different patterns of symptoms, despite having a similar diagnosis. Homeopathic medicine provides a sophisticated methodology for individualizing treatment for each child.

The Story of Eric: A Great Kid and a Terror

Eric was a nine-year-old whose father brought him to a homeopath because he had recurrent abdominal pain with nausea. Although Eric also had serious behavioral problems, the father did not imagine that homeopathy could do much for that and hoped that homeopathy could at least help Eric's abdominal condition.

Eric described his abdominal discomfort as a "knotlike pain" that was worse in the morning, especially upon waking. The pain returned when he got into bed at night. He also experienced it when he had to go somewhere he did not want to go, such as school. Sometimes he experienced the pain when getting ready to go somewhere he was excited about.

Eric said that the pain would be relieved when he could vomit. It was also somewhat relieved by soda pop and lying on his stomach.

Eric got frequent colds, though they were primarily a nasal obstruction rather than the runny type. His father noted that he always seemed to have this nasal obstruction. When his nose ran, it was usually yellow and got worse at night. He tended to cough when he woke up in the morning. He had leg pains in bed at night from the age of six, but this pain was relieved by warm baths.

Eric's other characteristic symptoms included a strong desire for open air, especially at night. He slept with lots of covers on, but insisted on having an open window. During the night, he often stuck his feet out of the covers or kicked them off. He preferred sleeping in a cool room.

Eric had a big appetite, though he was averse to anchovies, cooked vegetables, sardines, and fat. He craved garlic, sometimes eating an entire clove or eating garlic powder straight out of the jar. He also craved onions and yogurt.

Besides these physical characteristics, Eric had some disturbing emotional problems. His teacher described him as "a discipline problem" because he talked back to her, was extremely restless in class, had difficulty focusing, and continually "socialized" with kids during class. Although Eric was relatively bright, he was lazy and rarely did his homework. He also had problems with spelling and tended to write letters backwards (such as *q* for *p*). When out of the classroom, Eric got into lots of fights, often the result of telling someone to shut up.

One other noteworthy characteristic of Eric's personality was that he was a very messy boy, never cleaning or organizing his room unless forced to do so.

Eric was given a single dose of *Sulphur 30.* During the car ride home, he experienced one of his stomachaches. For the next month, he had a "cold," though this one was primarily of the runny type, not simply obstructive. During this month, he noticed that he was experiencing his stomach pains less and less often, until the pains occurred only very rarely. Of greatest significance (according to his parents and his teacher), Eric seemed a lot calmer. The teacher, who did not know that Eric had received a homeopathic medicine, mentioned to Eric's parents that he had changed dramatically for the better. Eric was not so restless, was not disturbing the class, and was not getting into fights.

It should be noted that the temporary exacerbation of stomach or other pains shortly after taking a homeopathic medicine is relatively common. The fact that Eric's chronic nasal obstruction was changed into a heavy nasal discharge was, from a homeopathic point of view, a direct effect of the body's curative effort to eliminate respiratory obstruction. Though this nasal discharge was irritating, it was recommended that nothing be done to stop it, since it was a part of the healing process. There is an adage that states: "Don't cure a cold, let a cold cure you." In this case, the adage was appropriate.

Besides the various improvements in Eric's physical and psychological health, his parents also noted that he was a lot more loving to them and to his baby sister. Despite all these impressive changes, they still bemoaned the fact that his room remained chronically messy.

Homeopathic medicines have wide applications for pediatric complaints. Since conventional medications, taken singularly or in combination with other drugs, have known and unknown complications in infants and children, it is generally worthwhile to seek safe, effective alternatives to pediatric problems first. Homeopathic medicines may not only help to improve the health of infants and children, but will probably also help them to become healthy adults.

Notes

1. Harris L. Coulter, *Divided Legacy: The Conflict Between Homoeopathy and the American Medical Association*, vol. 3 (Berkeley: North Atlantic Books, 1973), p. 71.

2. "General Guidelines for the Valuation of Drugs to Be Approved for Use During Pregnancy and for Treatment of Infants and Children," A Report of the Committee on Drugs, American Academy of Pediatrics, 1974.

3. Clinical Pharmacology Unit, University of Vermont College of Medicine, "Misuse of Antibiotics for Treatment of Upper Respiratory Infections in Children," *Pediatrics for the Clinician*, 1975.

4. Robert Mendelsohn, *How to Raise a Healthy Child . . . In Spite of Your Doctor* (Chicago: Contemporary Books, 1984), p. 13.

5. Wayne A. Ray et al., "Prescribing of Tetracycline to Children Less than 8 Years Old," *Journal of the American Medical Association*, 237 (1977): 2069–74.

6. Annabel Hecht, "What's That Alcohol Doing in My Medicine?" *FDA Consumer*, 18 (1984): 12–16.

7. Coulter, *Divided Legacy*, vol. 3, p. 114.

8. John S. Haller, Jr., "Aconite: A Case Study in Doctrinal Conflict and the Meaning of Scientific Medicine," *Bulletin of the New York Academy of Medicine*, 60 (November 1984): 900.

9. Ibid., p. 898.

10. Karin B. Nelson and Jonas H. Ellenberg, "Prognosis in Children with Febrile Seizures," *Pediatrics*, May 1978; Barton D. Schmitt, "Fever Phobia," *American Journal of Diseases of Children*, February 1980, pp. 176–186.

11. Gilbert Simon and Marcia Cohen, *Parent's Pediatric Companion* (New York: Marrow, 1985), p. 163.

12. Mendelsohn, *Healthy Child*, p. 3.

Additional References

Graedon, Joe. *The People's Pharmacy*. New York: St. Martin's Press, 1985.

Pantell, R. H., J. F. Fries, and D. M. Vickery. *Taking Care of Your Child*. Reading, Mass.: Addison-Wesley, 1985.

6

Women's Health:
Treating, Not Mistreating,
A Woman's Body

"Too many wives of conventional physicians are going to homeopathic physicians," complained one doctor at the 1883 meeting of the American Medical Association. "And to make matters worse," he added, "they are taking their children to homeopaths too!"[1]

Like the women of the 1800s, many of today's women have discovered that conventional medical treatment for numerous common health problems creates more harm than benefit. Since women visit medical doctors considerably more often than do men, they experience much greater risk associated with receiving more drugs, more surgery, and more medical interventions of other kinds.

Sadly enough, when women complain about the side effects from the various drugs they are taking, too often they are given another prescription, usually a tranquilizer. Research has shown that doctors prescribe twice the quantity of drugs for women as for men for what would be considered similar psychological symptoms.[2] According to a federal report, women receive 71 percent of the antidepressants prescribed, 80 percent of the amphetamines, and 60 percent of the mind-altering drugs.[3]

Once again, homeopathic medicine offers a distinct alternative. Homeopathic medicines are considerably safer, and they are also prescribed in minimum numbers of doses so that a sick person does not have to be bothered by or obsessed with continual treatment. And of greatest importance, homeopaths find that their medicines are effective, sometimes dramatically effective, in treating a wide range of women's common health problems, including premenstrual syndrome (PMS) and various menstrual disorders, vaginitis, cystitis (bladder infection), ovarian cysts, uterine fibroids, breast conditions, and the various symptoms of menopause. Effective treatment for women with breast, uterine, or ovarian cancer has also been reported, including slowing, stopping, and sometimes reversing the pathological processes.

Homeopathy, of course, is not *always* effective in treating women with cancer or any other chronic disease. There are numerous factors that affect the possible positive or negative outcomes from treatment. One reason that homeopaths do not succeed even more often than they do is that chronically ill people typically do not seek homeopathic care until their condition has progressed too far for recovery to be possible. Despite the various limitations inherent in many therapeutic encounters, homeopaths and their patients are generally impressed with the beneficial results obtained from homeopathic care.

The Homeopathic Treatment of PMS and Cystitis

When seeking to prescribe a homeopathic medicine for a woman, a homeopath always places special value on the symptoms of the reproductive system. The health of the reproductive system is a direct reflection of the delicate and dynamic interplay and balance between the hormonal and nervous systems, two of the most central regulatory mechanisms of the body.

To adjust hormonal imbalances, gynecologists commonly prescribe hormonal drugs such as birth control pills (sometimes prescribed to treat teenage acne), estrogens, progesterones, and synthetic male hormones. These drugs create higher levels of hormones circulating in the blood and reduce the symptoms that result from their deficiency. These drugs do not, however, deal with the underlying disharmony that created the deficiency in the first place, nor do they help the body to regain its ability to self-regulate a hormonal balance.

Homeopaths avoid the use of hormonal drugs, since they tend

to cover up symptoms without restoring health. When symptoms are suppressed, it is more difficult for the homeopath to select the appropriate individual medicine, since the woman's new symptoms are not necessarily the symptoms of her disease but are the effects of a drug on her body. Worse still, the body must now fight off the drug effects as well as the disease process.

Current researchers have conjectured that hormone-like chemical messengers in the body, called prostaglandins, are responsible for premenstrual syndrome. But these scientists are once again confusing a symptom with its cause. The excess prostaglandins found in the body of a woman who is experiencing premenstrual syndrome may be only another symptom of her disease.

In addition to hormones, other conventional drugs are often prescribed that simply treat individual PMS symptoms. Diuretics, for example, are used to treat the swelling that women experience premenstrually. These diuretics, however, deplete the body's supply of potassium, causing muscle aches and cramps. Once again, this conventional medical treatment is only symptomatic, offering temporary relief at best, and too often causing side effects.

Premenstrual syndrome has only recently become recognized as a health disorder. Homeopaths think of the diagnosis of premenstrual syndrome as a "Johnny-come-lately" label, for homeopaths have recognized this syndrome since the inception of homeopathy. They did not assume that symptoms prior to menstruation were "all in the head," as did most conventional physicians. In fact, homeopaths have made use of the various subtle or severe physical and/or psychological monthly symptoms that women often experience in order to find the correct individually prescribed medicine for them. Homeopaths and their women patients generally are particularly impressed with the results the medicines offer.

Women can even sometimes treat themselves for the occasional acute symptoms of their premenstrual condition, though it is generally recommended that they seek professional homeopathic care if they have recurrent or particularly strong symptoms. While there are several homeopathic medicines that are effective in relieving symptoms of an acute PMS condition without side effects, there are other homeopathic medicines that work on a deeper level to diminish the recurrence of chronic symptoms and to raise the overall health of the woman.

Whether they suffer from cramps, headaches, swelling, psychological changes, or other common premenstrual symptoms, it is worthwhile to know that women do not simply have to endure this monthly pain and discomfort. Rather than simply trying to reduce the amount of prostaglandins in their bodies or mechanically adjusting their delicate hormonal balance, women with premenstrual syndrome are finding great benefit in using homeopathic medicines.

Some of the common medicines for the woman with occasional acute symptoms of PMS are *Belladonna* (deadly nightshade), *Magnesia phosphorica* (phosphate of magnesia), *Colocynthis* (bitter cucumber), *Cimicifuga* (black snakeroot), *Chamomilla* (chamomile), *Caulophyllum* (blue cohosh), *Pulsatilla* (windflower), *Lachesis (venom of the bushmaster)*, *Sepia* (cuttlefish), and *Natrum mur* (salt).

Magnesia phosphorica (also called *Mag phos*) and *Colocynthis* are the two most common homeopathic medicines for menstrual cramps. Although the symptoms that each effectively treats are similar, each medicine also has characteristic symptoms that differentiate it from the other. The symptoms of women who need *Mag phos* are cramping pains relieved primarily by warmth, though also helped by pressure and bending forward. The pains sometimes center in the uterus and radiate in all directions. *Colocynthis* has similar symptoms, though the woman will primarily find her pains lessened by bending forward and secondarily by warmth and pressure. Another distinction from the women who needs *Mag phos* is that the woman who needs *Colocynthis* will generally be more irritable and angry, feelings that may even have preceded the onset of menstrual cramps.

Women can learn to treat themselves for several other acute health problems. The homeopathic literature is replete, for example, with stories of women treating themselves for a simple bladder infection. Strangely enough, one of the most common medicines for this condition is *Cantharis* (Spanish fly). Spanish fly is known as an aphrodisiac, but its actual effects on the body are that it creates such burning and irritation in the urinary tract that a woman wants her sexual organs touched and rubbed. It also creates great burning pain upon and after urination, which is also the primary symptom of the bladder infection. Because of this, homeopaths use microdoses of *Cantharis* to treat bladder infections effectively. Other common medicines given for bladder infections are *Sarsaparilla* (wild liquorice), *Mercurius* (mercury), *Nux vomica* (poison nut), *Berberis* (barberry), *Pulsatilla* (windflower), and *Apis* (crushed bee).

Conventional medicine offers antibiotics for bladder infections. Although these drugs seem to "work" (the infection disappears), 15 percent of all women get repeated bladder infections. It is generally recognized that, at best, antibiotics temporarily relieve a woman's infection and do not affect the factors that led to the infection. Ideally, it should be the goal of medicine to offer treatment that not only cures but strengthens the body sufficiently to prevent future problems. This is the often achieved goal of homeopathy.

The Homeopathic Treatment of Vaginal Infections and Chronic Problems

The value of homeopathy in treating various infectious diseases is also evidenced in its success in treating many women's infections. Vaginitis (inflammation or infection of the vagina) is a very common women's health problem. Various organisms may be associated with the infection, including *Candida albicans* (yeast), *Gardnerella* (previously called *Hemophilus*), *Trichomonas*, and *Chlamydia*.

In the coming years, modern medicine will no doubt discover other infectious organisms in women's vaginas, which will then be diagnosed as causing their own set of symptoms. Conventional drugs will inevitably be found to rid the body of these organisms, though, as discussed in the chapter on infectious disease (Chapter 7), these treatments will not necessarily cure the underlying disease or susceptibility to it. The use of conventional drugs will also eventually create drug-resistant organisms, and the drugs will each have their attendant side effects.

Rather than use medicines that attack a specific microorganism that has infected the body, the homeopath attempts to find the medicine that would stimulate the body's own immune and defense systems to rid itself of the infectious agent. A homeopathic medicine is individually prescribed based on an analysis of a woman's unique constellation of physical, emotional, and mental characteristics. To the homeopath, it is not so important to know what *microorganism* has infected the woman as it is to know *what kind of woman* the microorganism has infected. This homeopathic approach is a model of what Sir William Osler, the "father" of modern medicine, intended when he asserted: "Ask not what kind of illness the patient has, ask what kind of patient has the illness."

From this perspective, it is understandable that there are a select number of homeopathic medicines frequently given to women, depending on their individual typologies. Three of the most commonly prescribed medicines for women are not just for various acute infections but for various chronic health problems. These medicines are *Pulsatilla*, *Sepia*, and *Natrum mur.*

Just because a woman fits into one of these typologies does not necessarily mean that this medicine will cure all her ills or that no other homeopathic medicines will ever be prescribed. It does, however, mean that this particular medicine may be of particular importance in raising her level of health in a significant way, now and perhaps in the future as well.

Before describing the three common medicines and the attendant psychological and physical states they each treat, it should be mentioned that homeopaths do not assume that a woman will have *all* the symptoms of a single medicine. Instead, it is more common to find that a woman fits the *general* characteristics of a medicine. Homeopaths also find that once a homeopathic medicine works to improve the woman's overall level of health, another medicine may be indicated to further the healing process.

It should also be noted that homeopathic medicines are prescribed based on symptoms of disease or limitation of function, not on characteristics of health. Thus, the descriptions of the following three medicines and the types of women they are effective in treating primarily focus on the women's problems and weaknesses, rather than their strengths.

The women who need *Pulsatilla* are gentle, mild, and yielding. They are agreeable people who avoid quarrels, are sensitive to others' feelings, and are not aggressive. They are greedy for affection, approval, and sympathy, and are emotionally dependent on others. One of their greatest fears is of being abandoned. These women are moody, feeling happy at one moment and sad the next. They are quite emotional in general and are easily brought to tears, especially just prior to menstruation. Whether they are educated or not, *Pulsatilla* women rely on feelings in making decisions. With their changing moods, they are very indecisive, whether it be in relation to what they should eat, what they should wear, what college they should attend, what job they should have, or what they should do for entertainment. Being sweet and adaptable, *Pulsatilla* women see value in all their various choices, often making decisions by default or by taking another's advice. *Pulsatilla* women are easily led by others and easily hurt, too.

Physically, women who need *Pulsatilla* are generally "warm-blooded" (in homeopathic termology, "warm-blooded" means that a person is physically warmer than others and requires less clothing; a person who is "cold-blooded" gets cold easily and requires more clothing), dislike warm rooms, crave open air (their physical symptoms may even diminish when they are outside), and have unstable circulation (they flush and blush easily). Like their changing emotional state, their physical symptoms also drift, moving from one part of the body to another. *Pulsatilla* women are averse to eating fat (and sometimes will develop symptoms from it) and are also averse to warm food and drinks. Although they often have a dry mouth, they are thirstless.*

In contrast to women who need *Pulsatilla* are women who need *Sepia* (cuttlefish—a member of the mollusk family, which

---

*The "bodymind personalities" of the homeopathic medicines are often poetically described. Catherine Coulter's *Portraits of Homoeopathic Medicines* (Berkeley: North Atlantic Books, 1986) provides vivid descriptions of nine key medicines, including *Pulsatilla*. Besides discussing each medicine, Coulter also describes the root substance, how it grows and acts in nature, and how these characteristics correspond to the person who needs the medicine. Coulter notes that *Pulsatilla* (the herb "windflower") is a small and delicate flower with a flexible stem that moves with the wind (moody, easily "taken into the wind"). It grows in clusters (dependence on others) in dry, sandy soil (thirstlessness).

also includes clams, oysters, mussels, and snails). *Sepia* women are often overworked housewives or assertive career women. They are generally outspoken, direct, industrious, critical, and have a sense of duty. They are proudly independent and constantly strive for self-expression. However, they often keep things to themselves, even though they may feel great dissatisfaction. An inner irritability creates a bossy and nagging personality. They become fault-finding, discontent with everything, easily offended, and disposed to quarrel. They sometimes view love as a responsibility, a duty. They do not enjoy sex as much as other women. They may feel irritable after sex, may have a low sex drive, or may simply become averse to sex. They may also become indifferent to their husbands and even to their children.

Physically, *Sepia* women generally have low energy, are constipated, and sometimes are so "cold-blooded" that they may even feel cold in a warm room. Modern diagnostic procedures have found that *Sepia* women tend to have low thyroid hormones, low blood pressure, and adrenal deficiency. They often complain of a general "dragged-out feeling." They may describe experiencing an empty sensation in the mid-abdomen that is not relieved by eating. They tend to crave vinegar, acids, pickles, and sweets, but are averse to fat. Despite their low energy, they find obvious improvement in their physical and psychological state after exercise. They may have a sallow, bloated complexion. Other common symptoms include weakness in the small of the back and headaches.

The women who need *Natrum mur* (salt) are warm-blooded like *Pulsatilla* women and self-reliant like *Sepia* women, but they are unique in other ways. Probably their most prominent characteristic is their tendency to suffer from grief. Whether it be grief precipitated by a parent, a lover, or a close friend, women who need *Natrum mur* do not easily get over whatever past pain they have experienced. They retain it, allow it to fester and grow, and ultimately bear a longtime grudge against the person presumed to be responsible for it. No matter what the problem is, their self-reliant tendency prevents them from seeking any type of assistance; they are averse to any kind of sympathy. Their fierce independence may help them to develop special professional, artistic, or other skills, but it also keeps others from getting to know them. *Natrum mur* women are also very sensitive to any criticism or ridicule.

Because of the pain they experience, they have difficulty expressing affection or staying physically close to others. They become joyless, sad, and dejected. They take everything very seriously, viewing life as a duty and a responsibility that is full of sacrifices. They will only cry when alone, except when they cannot hold in their grief any longer, at which time they weep with uncontrollable sobbing. One way that women who need *Natrum mur* deal with their own grief is to help others as an advice-giver, counselor/therapist, teacher, missionary, lawyer, or doctor. They help others to attain the happiness that they themselves cannot have. They also have a strong sense of justice and hate things that are not fair. They will sacrifice themselves for a cause, whether it be political, religious, or artistic.

Physically, women who need *Natrum mur* have dry mucous membranes (mouth, vagina), oily skin (especially on the face), constipation, and general weakness and weariness (especially around 10 A. M.). Although they are warm-blooded and often need few clothes, they feel uncomfortable in hot sun, warm rooms, and heat in general. They are oversensitive to light, smoke, and noise, which make them irritable. Their symptoms are sometimes worse after eating, and they feel noticeably better when fasting. (*Natrum mur* is a common medicine for women who are anorexic, so long as their symptoms match the general picture of the medicine.) They do not sweat much, except occasionally while eating. At times they crave salt, bread, and bitter and sour substances, though at other times they can be averse to salt, bread, and any slimy foods, such as oysters or fat. They are prone to having profuse watery discharges when they have vaginitis or a common cold, and they are also prone to pressure headaches, especially from sunrise to sunset and before, during, and after menstruation. Modern diagnostic procedures find that women who need *Natrum mur* have hypoinsulinism, hypoadrenalism, and hyperthyroidism.

Each woman who has PMS, cystitis, vaginitis, or any other disease or condition may have symptoms in common with others, but there are always idiosyncratic symptoms or patterns of symptoms that are unique to the individual woman. The prescription of a homeopathic medicine based on this unique pattern helps to raise the overall health of the woman and ultimately helps to reduce or completely eliminate her symptoms of disease.

The Homeopathic Treatment of Menopause

Menopause, also called the "climacteric" or "the change of life," refers to the time in a woman's life, usually between the ages of 48 and 55, when she stops menstruating. The woman's ovaries decrease their production of estrogen, and her body adapts to the attendant changes. Common symptoms of menopause are hot flashes or flushes, a dry vagina, osteoporosis (a decrease in bone density), and perspiration. Although some women experience severe symptoms during this time of life, the vast majority notice little or no symptoms. Thus, the symptoms of menopause described here must not be thought of as a "normal" process but rather are representative of an unhealthy state.

Some of the most commonly prescribed drugs in medicine today are hormonal drugs given to women at and after menopause. The conventional treatment has been "Estrogen Replacement Therapy," whereby women are given female hormones to replace those that their bodies no longer produce. For several years, physicians were giving only estrogen. This treatment was controversial, however, because some studies found that estrogen's use led to an increased chance of uterine (endometrial) cancer. Recent studies have found that adding progestin, a synthetic form of progesterone (another female hormone), may reduce the risk of cancer, but other studies have found that this new combination drug carries the same risks of increasing incidence of cancer as other hormonal drugs.[4]

Since women who take Estrogen Replacement Therapy are expected to take the drugs throughout the rest of their lives, it seems that side effects are inevitable. Though recent research has evaluated the effects of these medicines after three or five years, it is anybody's guess what effects they will have after ten or twenty years. The question ultimately becomes: are the risks worth the benefits? Certainly, if conventional medicine offered the sole treatment for this condition, many women would probably conclude that the new estogen-progestin drug is worth the risks. However, there is some evidence that basic improvements in diet (increased amounts of calcium, vitamins C, D, and E, and bioflavonoids) and lifestyle changes (increased exercise) may be adequate in relieving most, if not all, symptoms of menopause.[5]

As for homeopathy, there has not yet been any good double-blind research confirming its value in treating women who are experiencing symptoms of menopause. However, there is pragmatic clinical experience that shows relief of these symptoms when homeopathic medicines are utilized.

Two of the three medicines commonly prescribed for women who are experiencing symptoms of menopause have already been discussed: *Sepia* and *Natrum mur.* The other commonly used medicine is *Lachesis* (venom of the bushmaster, a South American snake). The women who need *Lachesis* are generally energetic, loquacious, intense, and mistrustful of others. They are a very jealous type who commonly experience strong feelings of envy and hatred, though they go to great extents to suppress these feelings. There is an underlying resentment under the controlled surface. They are irritable, even at the slightest cause, and like the snake from which the medicine derives, they will strike back at the least provocation. They feel passionate about things, and because of this they tend to interrupt others in conversation, though they hate being interrupted themselves. They are fast thinking and talking and are quick-witted, though their humor is often malicious. They are very loyal to their friends and lovers, and they *demand* the same from others. Most often these women have strong sexual desires.

Physically, the women who need *Lachesis* tend to feel the worst physically and psychologically immediately upon waking in the morning. Their symptoms are also aggravated by heat and are often diminished by cold bathing or being in cold weather. They are very sensitive to pressure and do not like tight clothing, especially around the neck and abdomen. Many of their symptoms are manifested on the left side. They may crave alcohol, though they are sensitive to it, with a tendency to get headaches, heart palpitations, or other symptoms.

Lachesis is one of the most common medicines given to older women who have had health problems that began after their menopause—though, as always, homeopathic medicines must be individually prescribed.

Other common medicines for women who experience symptoms of menopause are *Calcarea carbonica*, *Sulphur*, and, less frequently, *Apis*, *Graphities*, *Phosphorus*, and *Psorinum*.

The late Elizabeth Wright Hubbard, M.D., a New York homeopathic physician, reported such good results in treating women with homeopathic medicines that she proclaimed: "Under homeopathy, life can begin at 60!"[6]

Notes

1. Harris L. Coulter, *Divided Legacy: The Conflict Between Homeopathy and the American Medical Association*, vol. 3 (Berkeley: North Atlantic Books, 1973), p. 116.

2. Robert S. Mendelsohn, *Male Practice: How Doctors Manipulate Women* (Chicago: Contemporary Books, 1982), p. 60.

3. Ibid.

4. Editors of Prevention Magazine, *Using Medicines Wisely* (Emmaus, Pa.: Rodale, 1985), pp. 94–96.

5. Ibid., p. 95.

6. Elizabeth Wright Hubbard, "Homeopathy During the Menopause," *Journal of the American Institute of Homeopathy*, 54 (March–April 1961): 45–46.

Additional References

Keyser, Herbert H. *Women Under the Knife*. New York: Warner, 1984.
Rosenfeld, Isadore. *Second Opinion*. New York: Bantam, 1982.
Smith, Trevor. *A Woman's Guide to Homoeopathic Medicine*. Wellingborough, England: Thorsons, 1984.
Weiss, Kay, ed. *Women's Health Care: A Guide to Alternatives*. Reston, Va.: Reston, 1984.

7

Infectious Disease: Effective Alternatives to Antibiotics

Toward the end of Louis Pasteur's life, he confessed that germs may not be the cause of disease after all, but may simply be another *symptom* of disease. He had come to realize that germs lead to illness primarily when the person's immune and defense systems (what biologists call "host resistance") are not strong enough to combat them. The "cause" of disease is not simply a bacterium or virus but also the factors that compromise host resistance, including the person's hereditary endowment, his nutritional state, the stresses in his life, and his psychological state. In describing one of his experiments with silkworms, Pasteur asserted that the microorganisms present in such large numbers in the intestinal tracts of the silkworms were "more an effect than a cause of disease."[1]

With these far-reaching insights, Pasteur conceived an ecological understanding of infectious disease. Infectious disease does not simply have a single cause but is the result of a complex web of interactions inside and outside the individual.

The Homeopathic and Ecological View of Infectious Disease

An analogy to help develop an understanding of the ecological perspective of infectious disease can be developed from the situa-

119

tion of mosquitoes and swamps. It is commonly known that mosquitoes infest swamps because swamps provide the still waters necessary for the mosquitoes to lay their eggs and for the eggs to hatch without disruption. In essence, swamps are a perfect environment for the mosquitoes to reproduce in.

A farmer might try to rid his land of mosquitoes by spraying insecticide over the swamps. If lucky, he will kill all the mosquitoes. However, because the swamp is still a swamp, it is still a perfect environment for new mosquitoes to fly in and lay their eggs. The farmer then sprays his insecticide again, only to find that more mosquitoes infest the swamp. Over time, some mosquitoes do not get sprayed with fatal doses of the insecticide. Instead, they adapt to the insecticide that they have ingested, and with each generation they are able to pass on to their offspring an increased immunity to the insecticide. Soon, the farmer must use stronger and stronger varieties of insecticide; but as the result of their adaptation, some mosquitoes are able to survive, despite exposure to the insecticide.

Similarly, finding streptococcus in a child's throat does not necessarily mean that the strep "caused" a sore throat, any more than one could say that the swamp "caused" the mosquitoes. Streptococcus often inhabits the throats of healthy people without leading to sore throats. Symptoms of strep throat only begin if there are favorable conditions for the strep to reproduce rapidly and to aggressively invade the throat tissue. Strep, like mosquitoes, will only settle and grow in conditions that are conducive for it.

The child with strep throat generally gets treated with antibiotics. Although the antibiotics may be effective in getting rid of the bacteria temporarily, they do not change the factors that led to the infection in the first place. When the farmer sprays with insecticide or the physician prescribes antibiotics but does not change the conditions that created the problem, the mosquitoes and the bacteria are able to return to those environments that are favorable for their growth.

To make matters worse, the antibiotics kill the beneficial bacteria along with the harmful ones. Since the beneficial bacteria play an important role in digestion, the individual's ability to assimilate necessary nutrients is temporarily limited, ultimately making him more prone to reinfection or other illness in the meantime.

Marc Lappé, a professor of public health and pharmacology at the University of Illinois and the author of *When Antibiotics Fail*, notes that "when these more benevolent counterparts die off, they leave behind a literal wasteland of vacant tissue and organs. These sites, previously occupied with normal bacteria, are now free to be colonized with new ones. Some of these new ones have caused serious and previously unrecognized diseases."[2]

Some clinicians have found that inappropriate antibiotic usage can transform common vaginal "yeast" infections *(candida albicans)*, which are characterized by simple itching, into a system-wide *candida* infection that can cause a variety of acute and chronic problems.[3] Although the diagnosis of "systemic candidaisis" is controversial, there is a consensus that frequent use of antibiotics can transform bacteria that normally live in our bodies without creating any problems into irritating and occasionally serious infections in the elderly, the infirm, and the immunodepressed.[4]

And, of course, bacteria learn to adapt to and survive antibiotics. Scientists then must either slightly change the antibiotics (there are over 300 varieties of penicillin alone) or make stronger and stronger antibiotics (which generally also have more and more serious side effects). Despite the best efforts of scientists, Dr. Lappé asserts that we are creating many more germs than medicines to fight them, since each new antibiotic brings to life literally millions of Benedict Arnolds.

Just fifteen to twenty years ago, penicillin was virtually always successful in treating gonorrhea. Now there are gonorrhea bacteria that have learned to resist penicillin, and these bacteria have now been found in all fifty states as well as throughout the world. From 1983 to 1984 alone, the number of cases in the United States with resistant strains of gonorrhea doubled.[5]

Alexander Fleming, the scientist who discovered penicillin, cautioned against the overuse of antibiotics. Unless the scientific community and the general public heed his warning, Harvard professor Walter Gilbert, a Nobel Prize–winner in chemistry, has asserted, "there may be a time down the road when 80 percent to 90 percent of infections will be resistant to all known antibiotics."[6]

The scientific community and the general public need to pay

more attention to Pasteur's insights and the importance of host resistance in preventing illness. Most scientists have broadly accepted
the germ theory, whereas only rare individuals have acknowledged
the importance of the ecological balance of microorganisms in the
body. But the wisdom of Pasteur remains relevant, and more and
more scientists are beginning to acknowledge the importance of
alternatives to antibiotics. Even an editorial in the prestigious *New
England Journal of Medicine* has affirmed the need for the treatment of infections with "less ecologically disturbing techniques."[7]
Homeopathic medicines will inevitably play a major role as one
of these alternatives.

Are Antibiotics Helpful in Ear and Throat Infections?

Claude Bernard, the esteemed "father of experimental physiology,"
affirmed Pasteur's contention that bacteria are not the cause of
disease. In one of his most famous books, Bernard noted that if
the exciting cause were the principal factor—for instance, in pneumonia—everyone exposed to cold would come down with this
disease, whereas only an occasional case of chill turns into pneumonia. He concluded that unless the subject is predisposed, the
most powerful causes will have no effect on him. He therefore
asserted that predisposition is the "pivot of all experimental physiology" and the real cause of most disease.[8]

At a health conference in 1976, Jonas Salk noted that there
are basically two ways to heal sick people. First, one can try to
control the individual symptoms that the sick person is experiencing; and second, one can try to stimulate the person's own immune and defense systems to enable the body to heal itself.[9] Whereas conventional medicine's allegiance is to the first approach,
homeopathy and a wide variety of natural healing systems attempt
the latter.

A good example of the questionable value of the use of antibiotics is their application in children's earaches. Ear infection
has become one of the most common childhood illnesses. The infection of the middle ear and eardrum is called "otitis media,"

a condition for which most physicians prescribe antibiotics. Several researchers, however, have found that antibiotics do not improve the health of children compared to that of children who are not given antibiotics.[10] Other researchers have found that antibiotics provide a brief relief of symptoms, but that subsequently there is no difference in these children from those given a placebo.[11] Still other researchers have found that 70 percent of children with otitis media still have fluid in their ears after four weeks of treatment and that 50 percent of children experience another ear infection within three months.[12]

Although some physicians assert that antibiotics are responsible for the presently low incidence of complications from ear infections such as mastoiditis, research has shown that there is no evidence that antibiotics reduce the incidence of mastoiditis.[13] Homeopaths claim a similarly low complication rate without the use of antibiotics.[14]

One of the more significant studies showed that patients with ear infections who were treated with antibiotics had appreciably more recurrence (as much as 2.9 times) than patients who did not use any treatment.[15]

In chronic ear infections, it has become standard procedure for physicians to use ear tubes in conjunction with or in place of antibiotics. These tubes help to drain the pus from the ear, but this treatment only deals with the results of the problem; it does nothing to treat the reason the infection was able to spread in the first place. This physiological fact may be the reason that ear tubes have been found to be of questionable value.[16]

Antibiotics and ear tubes treat the symptoms of a problem. They do not strengthen the organism so that it can fight the infection itself, nor do they make the organism more resistant to future infection.

Another myth that continues to be perpetuated is that of the value of antibiotics in treating sore throats. The primary rationale for using antibiotics to treat a sore throat has been to prevent the person from getting rheumatic fever, a potentially fatal condition. Researchers point out that there is presently an extremely low incidence of rheumatic fever. This low incidence, however, is not the result of antibiotic use, because there was a decrease in rheumatic fever incidence even prior to antibiotic use.*

Recent research has even determined that today's strains of streptococcus very rarely cause rheumatic fever,[17] and that antibiotics do not even eradicate the strep in 25–40 percent of the cases, despite the demonstrated sensitivity of the organism to the antibiotic.[18]

Also, it is widely recognized that most strep infections are left untreated, and yet a vast majority of these people do not get rheumatic fever. Furthermore, from 33 to 50 percent of the cases of rheumatic fever occur without sore throat symptoms.[19] A recent outbreak of rheumatic fever was reported in the *New England Journal of Medicine*.[20] Two-thirds of the children with this disease had no clear-cut history of a sore throat within a three-month period preceding the onset of their condition. Of particular significance is the fact that of the eleven children who had throat symptoms and who thus had a throat culture performed, eight tested positive for strep. These children were prescribed antibiotics, and yet each still developed rheumatic fever.

New evidence shows that antibiotics do help to reduce the

---

*See Alan L. Bisno, "Where Has All the Rheumatic Fever Gone?" *Clinical Pediatrics*, December 1983, pp. 804–805; and M. Land, "Acute Rheumatic Fever: A Vanishing Disease in Suburbia," *Journal of the American Medical Association*, 249 (1983): 895–898. In 1986, there were some reports of new outbreaks of rheumatic fever in some parts of the United States. However, Ellen Wald, M.D., medical director of Children's Hospital of Pittsburgh, noted that too-early treatment with antibiotics may impair the body's normal immunologic response and open up the possibility of reinfection, and that this problem must be weighed against the benefit of possibly preventing rheumatic fever. One recent study has shown that those children who were treated with antibiotics immediately upon diagnosis had eight times the recurrent rate of strep throat compared to those children who delayed treatment ("Pediatricians Urge Confirmatory Test for Suspected Strep Throat," *Medical World News*, January 12, 1987, p. 42). In the context of other studies cited in this chapter, it may be worthwhile to compare children who received delayed treatment with those who received no antibiotics. It may also be worthwhile to compare these groups with a group of children prescribed a homeopathic medicine.

symptoms of sore throat faster than placebos.[21] However, it is questionable if antibiotics should be used simply to relieve self-limited conditions. It is certainly understandable that antibiotic use be considered when there is a life-threatening condition. However, it is uncertain how effective they are in preventing one rare disease. It is also uncertain if it is worth prescribing these powerful drugs to mass numbers of children in the hope that a very small number *might* benefit.

Antibiotics should definitely not be given routinely to children with *suspected* strep throat. Recent research has shown that 60 percent of children's sore throats are caused by viruses, for which antibiotics are useless.[22]

This evidence strongly suggests that alternatives to antibiotic usage should be sought for ear and throat infections. Homeopathy offers a viable alternative.

The Homeopathic Treatment of Infectious Disease

When people think about the successes of modern medicine, they often assert that we are now living considerably longer than our parents or grandparents. They also usually point to modern medicine's successes in treating the infectious diseases that raged during previous centuries, such as the plague, cholera, scarlet fever, yellow fever, and typhoid.

Scientists and historians alike agree that these assumptions are pure myths. Scientists point out that we are now living longer than ever before, but this has not primarily been the result of new medical technologies. Rather, our lengthening life is mostly attributable to (1) a significant decrease in infant mortality, which is the result of better hygiene during birth (hurray for soap!), (2) better nutrition (the creation of cities has enabled more people to have access to a greater variety of foods, thereby decreasing malnutrition), and (3) improvements in various public health measures such as sanitation, better sewage, cleaner water, and pest control.[23]

Even with all these considerations, the increase in life expectancy for adults has not been very significant. Statistics show that the average white male who reached 40 years of age in 1960 can expect to live to be 71.9; whereas the average white male who reached 40 years of age in 1920 lived to be 69.9. The average white male who reached 50 years of age in 1982 can expect to live to be 75.6; whereas the average white male who reached 50 years of age in 1912 lived to be 72.2 years.[24]

Pulitzer Prize-winning microbiologist René Dubos noted that "the life expectancy of adults is not very different now from what it was a few generations ago, nor is it greater in areas where medical services are highly developed than in less prosperous countries."[25]

Historians and epidemiologists remind us that conventional medicine was not at all responsible for the disappearance of or decrease in the fatal infectious diseases of the 15th to 19th centuries.[26] Antibiotics were not even available until the 1940s, and no other conventional drugs were successfully used to treat most of the epidemics of the past. Even mortality (incidence of death) from tuberculosis, pneumonia, bronchitis, influenza, and whooping cough was on a sharp decline prior to the introduction of any conventional medical treatment for them. An important exception was the decrease in the death rate from polio after the introduction of the polio vaccine.

A little-known fact of history is that homeopathic medicine developed its popularity in both the United States and Europe because of its successes in treating epidemics that raged during the 19th century. Dr. Thomas L. Bradford's *The Logic of Figures*, published in 1900, compares in detail the death rates in homeopathic versus allopathic (conventional) medical hospitals and shows that the death rate per 100 patients in homeopathic hospitals was often one-half or even one-eighth that of conventional medical hospitals.[27]

In 1849, the homeopaths of Cincinnati claimed that in over a thousand cases of cholera only 3 percent of the patients died. To substantiate their results, they even printed in a newspaper the names and addresses of patients who died or survived.[28] The death rate of cholera patients who used conventional medicines generally ranged from 40 to 70 percent.

The success of treating yellow fever with homeopathy was

so impressive that a report from the United States Government's Board of Experts discussed the value of several homeopathic medicines, despite the fact that the Board was primarily composed of conventional physicians who despised homeopathy.[29]

The success of homeopathy in treating modern-day infections is comparable to its successes in treating the infectious diseases of the last century. It is common knowledge that homeopathic practitioners rarely resort to using antibiotics or other drugs commonly given for infectious conditions. Homeopaths, like any good medical professional, will use antibiotics when clearly necessary, but it is worthwhile having alternatives that work.

Homeopath Randall Neustaedter of Palo Alto, California, notes that acute ear infection is "a simple problem to manage with acute [homeopathic] remedies."[30] Common acute ear infection medicines are *Belladonna* (deadly nightshade), *Chamomilla* (chamomille), *Pulsatilla* (windflower), *Ferrum phos* (phosphate of iron), and *Hepar sulph* (Hahnemann's calcium sulphide).

If a child is treated with antibiotics and then has recurrent ear infections, homeopathic treatment generally takes more time but is often curative. Such recurrent problems, Neustaedter asserts, require the homeopathic "constitutional approach," the approach whereby a homeopathic medicine is prescribed based on the totality of present symptoms as well as on an evaluation of the patient's past history. While it is common for parents to prescribe successfully for acute ear infections, it is recommended that children receive professional care for recurrent ear infections or for any chronic condition.

Homeopaths have also found great success in treating a wide variety of other bacterial infections. Throat infections are commonly treated with *Belladonna* (deadly nightshade), *Arsenicum* (arsenic), *Rhus tox* (poison ivy), *Mercurius* (mercury), *Hepar sulph* (Hahnemann's calcium sulphide), *Lachesis* (venom of the bushmaster), *Apis* (crushed bee), or *Phytolacca* (pokeroot). Boils that result from bacterial infection are often successfully treated with *Belladonna, Hepar sulph, Silica* (silica), *Arsenicum*, or *Lachesis*. And styes, which usually result from a *Staphylococcus* infection, are effectively treated with *Pulsatilla, Hepar sulph, Apis, Graphities* (graphite), and *Staphysagria* (stavesacre).

In addition to treating bacterial infections, there is evidence that suggests that the homeopathic microdoses can also prevent specific bacterial conditions. In an impressive study, 18,640 Brazilian children were given a single dose of *Meningococcin 10c* (a homeopathic preparation of Neisseria meningitidis). The immunized group had significantly fewer cases of meningitis than other children who lived in the same community.[31]

The Homeopathic Treatment of Viral Conditions

Conventional drugs at least relieve the symptoms of bacterial infection; however, there is little in conventional medicine to treat most viral conditions. Since homeopathic medicines stimulate the body's own defenses rather than directly attacking specific pathogens, homeopathy again has much to offer in the treatment of viral diseases.

In recent research on viruses that attack chicken embryos, eight of the ten homeopathic medicines tested inhibited the growth of the viruses 50 to 100 percent.[32] This research is of particular significance because conventional science knows only a very select number of drugs that have antiviral action, and none of these drugs is as safe as the homeopathic medicines.

Homeopaths commonly treat people suffering from acute and chronic viral conditions. People with viral respiratory and digestive conditions, viral infection of the nervous system, herpes, and even a few with AIDS have reported significant improvement using homeopathic medicines. Sometimes this improvement is dramatic and immediate, though most of the time there is a slow, progressive improvement in the person's overall health.

British physician Richard Savage notes that "while the search goes on to find specific antiviral preparations which are free from side effects, homeopathy can be used effectively to treat patients in four ways: (1) *prophylaxis* to generate resistance to the infection; (2) *treatment in the acute illness* to reduce the length and severity of the illness; (3) *restoration* to revitalize the patient during convalescence; and (4) *correction of the chronic sequelae* to restore the patient to his former state of health."[33] Let us consider these one at a time.

Prophylaxis

In the 1800s, homeopaths commonly used medicines to prevent or cure what later came to be understood as bacterial and viral infections. *Aconite* and *Ferrum phos* were frequently given at the early onset of fever and aches as a way to prevent influenza; *Belladonna* was the most common medicine for preventing or treating scarlet fever; and *Camphora* (camphor) was the major medicine used to prevent or treat cholera. The dramatic success of the medicines in the prevention and treatment of these dread diseases gained homeopathy a large following.

Homeopaths commonly find that successful treatment of acute or chronic disease with homeopathic medicines leads to stronger and healthier people who do not become severely or recurrently ill. During the late 1800s, many life insurance companies offered lower rates to people who went to homeopathic physicians, because actuarial statistics showed that homeopathic patients were healthier and lived longer.[34] There is also a record that these life insurance companies paid out larger sums of money to homeopathic patients, since they lived longer than those under conventional medical care.[35]

Treatment of Acute Illness

One of the additional advantages of using homeopathy in treating viral conditions is that homeopathic medicines can be prescribed even before a definitive diagnosis has been made. This is because homeopaths prescribe based on the totality of symptoms, and laboratory work is not always necessary to find the correct medicine. Since some viral conditions are difficult to diagnose even after laboratory tests, one is often able to cure people with homeopathy before a conventional medical diagnosis can be made.

Antibiotics are only helpful in certain bacterial infections, and since viral diseases are particularly common, conventional medicine offers little help. In comparison, homeopaths often successfully treat acute viral conditions such as the common cold, virus-induced coughs, influenza, gastroenteritis (sometimes called the "stomach flu"), and viral hepatitis.

Homeopaths use *Allium cepa* (onion), *Euphrasia* (eyebright), *Natrum mur* (salt), or other individually chosen medicines for the common cold. *Aconite* (monkshood), *Belladonna*, *Bryonia* (wild hops), *Phosphorus* (phosphorus), and others are helpful in treating common viral respiratory infections.

Influenza, a condition that results from viral infection, is easily treated with homeopathy. Although individualization of homeopathic medicines is generally a necessity in order for them to work, there are conditions in which certain medicines are particularly effective. *Oscillococcinum* (pronounced o-sill-o-cock-SIGH-num) is a medicine that homeopaths have found particularly effective in treating the flu. Its manufacturer, Boiron Laboratories of Lyon, France, has found that it is 80–90 percent effective in treating the flu when taken within forty-eight hours of the onset of symptoms. Its success is so widely known in France that it is the most widely used treatment for the flu in that country.

Interestingly enough, *Oscillococcinum* is a microdose of the heart and liver of a duck. One might easily wonder how such a substance could ever be beneficial for the flu, but there actually is some sound logic to it. Research at the Mayo Clinic has shown that chicken soup has some antiviral action. Since chicken soup is basically a broth of the organs of chickens, perhaps *Oscillococcinum* is effective because it is "duck soup."

Ben Hole, M.D., a practicing homeopath in Orinda, California, reports: "Oscillococcinum is impressively successful, but in the rare situations where it doesn't work or isn't available, there are several other homeopathic medicines which can be used with excellent results when they are individually prescribed."

Other commonly used homeopathic medicines for the flu include *Gelsemium* (yellow jasmine), *Bryonia*, *Rhus tox*, and *Eupatorium perfoliatum* (boneset).

Restoration from Recurrent or Long-lasting Viral Infection

Although conventional medicine offers very little relief for recurrent or long-lasting viral infections, homeopaths have observed that microdoses relieve the symptoms of various chronic viral conditions such as herpes simplex, herpes genitales, chronic Epstein-Barr virus, and warts. One cannot claim that homeopathic medicines actually "cure" these viral conditions, since the virus is assumed to remain in the body throughout one's life, though homeopaths find that their patients get significantly less severe bouts of infection or do not get any symptoms for long periods of time.

The homeopathic approach to treating all these disorders includes a thorough analysis of the person's totality of symptoms. There is thus no one medicine for a specific disease.

Correction of the Chronic Sequelae

After a viral (or even bacterial) infection, people sometimes feel that they are still not back to their former healthy self. Generally, an individually chosen homeopathic medicine is prescribed. If the individualized medicine does not work, homeopaths will occasionally give a potentized dose of the specific virus that previously infected the person as a way to strengthen his ability to regain health. *Varicellinum* (exudate from a chicken pox vesicle) is commonly given in a safe microdose for symptoms that linger after the chicken pox, and *Parotidinum* (exudate with mumps virus) is often given for symptoms that linger after the mumps.

For the post-herpetic neuralgias, the common medicines are *Hypericum* (St. John's Wort), *Kalmia* (mountain laurel), *Magnesia phosphorica* (phosphate of magnesia), *Causticum* (Hahnemann's potassium hydrate), *Mezereum* (spurge olive), or *Arsenicum.*

A state of weakness after a bout of influenza is often treated with *China* (cinchona bark), *Gelsemium, Sulphur* (sulphur), *Phosphoricum acidum* (phosphoric acid), *Cadmium* (cadmium), or *Avena sativa* (oat).

Respiratory infections occasionally linger, creating chronic nasal discharge, sinusitis, and ear infections. Some of the common medicines given are *Kali bichromium* (bichromate of potash), *Kali iodatum* (potassium iodide), *Kali carbonicum* (potassium carbonate), *Kali muriaticum* (Chloride of potassium), *Kali sulphuricum* (potassium sulphate), *Silicea* (silica), *Mercurius, Pulsatilla, Alumina* (aluminum), *Nux vomica* (poison nut), and *Conium* (hemlock).

The Homeopathic Perspective
on and Treatment of AIDS

AIDS, like any infectious disease, is thought to result from infection by a specific virus in a person whose immune and defense systems are not strong enough to combat it. It is presently estimated that between 20 and 50 percent of people who are exposed to the virus tend to get AIDS. One of the theories why some people have a greater risk of getting AIDS, once exposed, is called the "immune overload hypothesis."[36] This hypothesis conjectures that there may be numerous factors that weaken the immune system, including poor nutrition, repeated bacterial infections, previous viral infections, rectal intercourse, genetic predisposition, intravenous narcotic drugs, and recreational drug use (amyl nitrate, in particular, has been found to be immunosuppressive; marijuana and cocaine have immunosuppressive effects, too).

There is, however, one additional factor that scientists and journalists have ignored when considering co-factors to AIDS.* While many scientists and journalists have pointed their fingers at recreational drugs that weaken the immune system, they have ignored the fact that many commonly used therapeutic drugs do so also. There is, in fact, epidemiological and toxicological evidence to suggest that antibiotics, corticosteroids, and the smallpox vaccine may be additional co-factors in making someone susceptible to AIDS.

Epidemiological evidence indicates that AIDS originated in Central Africa not only from sexual practices but also, according to *Newsweek*, from "the practice among health workers in Africa of using a single needle to inject a number of patients with penicillin and other drugs."[37] Similar unhygienic use of needles is common in Haiti, where antibiotics are available over-the-counter and are often taken for all sorts of inappropriate nonbacterial diseases. At the same time that their bodies' ecology is being disrupted by the antibiotic, these people are getting exposed directly to the virus

---

*A co-factor is a contributing factor to a disease.

through the needle.

The primary risk groups for AIDS in the United States and Europe, gay men and intravenous drug users, are both major abusers of antibiotics. Significant numbers of gay men have used these drugs recurrently because of frequent exposure to venereal diseases or to parasites. Intravenous drug users also commonly use antibiotics because of the frequent infections they develop as a result of shared needles.

Strictly speaking, penicillin is not considered to be immunosuppressive, as are other antibiotics such as tetracycline and cyclosporin. There is, however, toxicological evidence that, in overdose (or in regular dose in sensitive individuals), penicillin and most other antibiotics cause a decrease in white blood cells, diarrhea with poor absorption of food and gradual loss of weight, decreased resistance to infection, skin rashes, persistent fever and chills, weakness and prostration, and disease of the nervous system—all of which are also primary symptoms of AIDS.[38]

It must be clarified that this evidence does not suggest that antibiotics "cause" AIDS, but, more precisely, that they may be an additional co-factor to it when a person has been exposed to the virus.

Antibiotics may not be the only therapeutic drugs that are co-factors to AIDS. Hans H. Neumann of the Connecticut Department of Health reported in the *New England Journal of Medicine* that corticosteroids may contribute to immunosuppression and thus increase the chances of getting AIDS if a person becomes infected with the virus. Neumann noted that some gay men have used over-the-counter cortisone creams for genital herpes and for skin irritations of the anal and genital areas. The thin penile skin is particularly suited for absorption of the cortisone, and anal sex leads to absorption of the cortisone by one's partner.[39]

A recent article in the *New England Journal of Medicine* has implicated the smallpox vaccine as another co-factor to AIDS.[40] New research has indicated that the smallpox vaccine may trigger a dormant AIDS virus into having immunosuppressive activity. The World Health Organization (WHO), which has a worldwide smallpox vaccination program, has begun to study this possible connection. An adviser to WHO told The *Times* (of London):

"Now I believe the smallpox vaccine theory is the explanation to the explosion of AIDS."[41] Even Dr. Robert Gallo, one of the most respected AIDS researchers, told The *Times:* "The link between the WHO program and the epidemic in Africa is an interesting and important hypothesis. I cannot say that it actually happened, but I have been saying for some years that the use of live vaccines such as that used for smallpox can activate a dormant infection such as HIV [Human Immunodeficiency Virus]."[42]

This evidence suggests that there may indeed by an iatrogenic (doctor-induced) side to AIDS. There are, no doubt, other stresses that play a more significant role in leading to AIDS for many people who are infected, but we must not ignore the possibility of various co-factors to this dread disease.

As for the homeopathic treatment of people with AIDS and with ARC (AIDS-related complex), there is general agreement that little can be done to help those individuals with end-stage AIDS. As for those who have recently been diagnosed with AIDS or ARC, several homeopaths have noted improvement in certain patients' general health and in their T-cell and B-cell counts (these are important indices for measuring the strength of the immune system).

As of mid-1987, there are approximately two hundred and fifty people with AIDS under homeopathic care. A systematic evaluation of these people will be under way when funding for the research is made available.

As for people who have been exposed to the virus but who have not developed AIDS, several homeopaths have observed that the use of homeopathic medicines may help strengthen people so that they do not become ill. Michael Strange, a London homeopath, has noted that he has forty-five patients who tested positive to the HIV antibody test for an average of two years, and thus far none has developed AIDS.[43]

Although each person with AIDS or ARC is treated individually, some of the more commonly used medicines are *Mercurius* (mercury), *Thuja* (arbor vitae), *Arsenicum* (arsenic), *Syphilinum* (exudate from syphilis chancre), *Tuberculinum* (tubercle bacilli), *Phosphorus* (phosphorus), *Calcarea phosphorica* (calcium phosphate), *Nitricum acid* (nitric acid), *Natrum mur* (salt), *Lachesis* (venom of the bushmaster), *Crotalus horridus* (venom of the rattlesnake), and *Variolinum* (exudate from a smallpox pustule). One researcher found that *Typhoidinum* (typhoid bacilli), *Badiaga* (freshwater sponge), and *Cyclosporin* (an antibiotic) were most commonly indicated.[44] It is logical that *Cyclosporin* (in homeopathic potency) may be a valuable medicine for people with AIDS, since this medicine in conventional dose is a known immunosuppressive drug, and thus in microdose it may be helpful to heal an immunosuppressive condition such as AIDS.

No carefully controlled research has yet definitely shown the efficacy of homeopathy in treating people with AIDS or ARC. However, the research previously mentioned showing the antiviral action of homeopathic medicines,[45] the study that proved the effectiveness of the homeopathic medicines in treating a different disease of the immune system (rheumatoid arthritis),[46] and the evidence that homeopathy was effective in treating previous major infectious diseases provide some evidence to suggest that it may be of value in treating people with AIDS or ARC. Research on the use of homeopathic medicine to treat people with AIDS or ARC holds promise and is worthy of funding.

In Conclusion

The homeopathic and ecological understanding of infectious disease is one that takes into account the factors in the body and the environment that make it possible for infection to take place and to spread. Rather than use treatments that attack bacteria or viruses, homeopaths use microdoses of the individually selected homeopathic medicine to strengthen the body's own immune and defense systems. Such treatment reduces the possibility of bacterial or viral spread and leads to regained health and vigor.

The famous Indian Chief Seattle once remarked: "We are part of the web of life. We are not the weaver. When a part of the web is destroyed, a part of ourselves is hurt." The bacteria and the viruses that are inside us are a part of us. Conventional medicines that try to get rid of them often create their own set of problems. It is perhaps no accident that the word *antibiotic* itself is derived from words that mean "anti-life." Although antibiotics can be real lifesavers, they tend to disrupt the complex web of life inside us. It is now clearer than ever that judicious use of antibiotics is a necessity. And it is becoming increasingly obvious that homeopathic medicines provide a viable, safer alternative to antibiotic use.

Notes

1. René Dubos, *Mirage of Health* (San Francisco: Harper and Row, 1959), pp. 93–94.

2. Marc Lappé, *When Antibiotics Fail* (Berkeley: North Atlantic Books, 1986), p. xii.

3. William Crook, *The Yeast Connection* (New York: Vintage, 1986).

4. Lappé, *When Antibiotics Fail*, p. xiii.

5. Ibid., p. xvii.

6. "Those Overworked Miracle Drugs," *Newsweek*, August 17, 1981, p. 63.

7. R. B. Sack, "Prophylactic Antibiotics? The Individual Versus the Community," *New England Journal of Medicine*, 300 (1979): 1107–08.

8. Claude Bernard, *Principes de Médecine Expérimentale* (Paris: Presses Universitaires de France, 1947), pp. 160–161.

9. Jonas Salk, Mandala Holistic Health Conference, San Diego, Calif., September 1976. Proceedings published in *Journal of Holistic Health*, 1976.

10. F. L. Von Buchem, "Therapy of Acute Otitis Media: Myringotomy, Antibiotics, or Neither? A Double-Blind Study in Children," *Lancet*, 883 (October 24, 1981): 883–887.

11. J. Thomsen, "Penicillin and Acute Otitis Media: Short and Long-term Results," *Annals of Otology, Rhinology, and Laryngology*, Supplement, 68 (1980): 271.

12. E. M. Mandel et al., "Efficacy of Amoxicillin with and without Decongestant—Antihistamine for Otitis Media with Effusion in Children," *New England Journal of Medicine*, 316 (February 19, 1987): 432–437.

13. Von Buchem, "Therapy," pp. 883–887.

14. Randall Neustaedter, "Management of Otitis Media with Effusion in Homeopathic Practice," *Journal of the American Institute of Homeopathy*, 79 (September–December 1986): 87–99, 133–140.

15. M. Diamant, "Abuse and Timing of Use of Antibiotics in Acute Otitis Media," *Archives of Otolaryngology*, 100 (1974): 226.

16. D. Kilby, "Grommets and Glue Ears: Two Year Results," *Journal of Laryngology and Otology*, 86 (1972): 105; M. J. K. M. Brown, "Grommets and Glue Ear: A Five-year Follow-up of a Controlled Trial," *Journal of Social Medicine*, 71 (1978): 353; T. Lildholdt, "Ventilation Tubes in Secretory Otitis Media," *Acta Otolaryngology*, Supplement, 398 (1983):1.

17. Alan L. Bisno, "Where Has All the Rheumatic Fever Gone?" *Clinical Pediatrics*, December 1983, pp. 804–805.

18. A. Gastanaduy, "Failure of Penicillin to Eradicate Group A Streptococci During an Outbreak of Pharyngitis," *Lancet*, 8193 (1980): 498–502; E. Kaplan, "The Role of the Carrier in Treatment Failures After Antibiotic Therapy for Group A Streptococci in the Upper Respiratory Tract," *Journal of Laboratory and Clinical Medicine*, 98 (1981): 326–335.

19. Alan L. Bisno, "The Concept of Rheumatogenic and Non-rheumatogenic Group A Streptococci," in Read, *Streptococcal Diseases and the Immune Response* (New York: Academic Press, 1980), pp. 789–803; Bisno, "Streptococcal Infections that Fail to Cause Recurrences of Rheumatic Fever," *Journal of Infectious Disease*, 136 (1977): 278–285.

20. A. George Veasy et al., "Resurgence of Acute Rheumatic Fever in the Intermountain Area of the United States," *New England Journal of Medicine*, 316 (February 19, 1987): 421–426.

21. James W. Bass, "Treatment of Streptococcal Pharyngitis," *Journal of the American Medical Association*, 256 (August 8, 1986): 740–743.

22. *Health Facts*, 12 (May 1987): 2.

23. René Dubos, *Mirage of Health* (New York: Harper and Row, 1959); Thomas McKeown, *The Role of Medicine* (Princeton: Princeton University Press, 1979).

24. "Life Tables," *Vital Statistics of the United States, 1982* (Hyattsville, Md.: National Center for Health Statistics, 1982), vol. 2, sec. 6, p. 13.

25. René Dubos, *Man Adapting* (New Haven: Yale University Press, 1965), p. 346.

26. McKeown, *Role of Medicine*, pp. 29–44.

27. Thomas L. Bradford, *The Logic of Figures or Comparative Results of Homoeopathic and Other Treatments* (Philadelphia: Boericke and Tafel, 1900).

28. Ibid., p. 68.

29. Harris L. Coulter, *Divided Legacy: The Conflict Between Homoeopathy and the American Medical Association*, vol. 3 (Berkeley:

North Atlantic Books, 1973), p. 302.

30. Neustaedter, "Management," p. 87.

31. David Castro and George Galvao Nogueira, "Use of the Nosode Meningococcinum as a Preventive Against Meningitis," *Journal of the American Institute of Homoeopathy*, 68 (December 1975): 211–219.

32. L. M. Singh and Girish Gupa, "Antiviral Efficacy of Homoeopathic Drugs Against Animal Viruses," *British Homoeopathic Journal*, 74 (July 1985): 168–174.

33. Richard Savage, "Homoeopathy: When No Effective Alternative," *British Homoeopathic Journal*, 73 (April 1984): 75–83.

34. *Transactions of the New York State Homoeopathic Medical Society*, 1867, pp. 57–59.

35. "Report of Life Insurance Committee," *Transactions of the American Institute of Homoeopathy*, 1897, pp. 53–58; 1898, pp. 81–90.

36. Victor Gong, *Understanding AIDS: A Comprehensive Guide* (New Brunswick, N.J.: Rutgers University Press, 1985), pp. 77–89.

37. Matt Clark et al., "AIDS," *Newsweek*, August 12, 1985, p. 22.

38. *Physicians' Desk Reference* (Oradell, N.J.: Medical Economics Books, 1985).

39. Hans H. Neumann, "Use of Steroid Creams as a Possible Cause of Immunosuppression in Homosexuals," *New England Journal of Medicine*, 306 (April 15, 1982): 935.

40. Robert R. Redfield et al., "Disseminated Vaccinia in a Military Recruit with Human Immunodeficiency Virus (HIV) Disease," *New England Journal of Medicine*, 316 (March 12, 1987): 673–676; Neal A. Halsey and D. A. Henderson, "HIV Infection and Immunization Against Other Agents," *New England Journal of Medicine*, 316 (March 12, 1987): 684–685.

41. Pearce Wright, "Smallpox Vaccine 'Triggered AIDS Virus,'" *The Times* (London), May 11, 1987, p. 1.

42. Ibid., p. 18.

43. Personal communication to the author. For additional information, see Michael Strange, "AIDS: What Homoeopathy Can Offer," *The Homoeopath: Journal of the Society of Homoeopaths*, 6 (1987): 117–124.

44. Laurence E. Badgley, "Homeopathy for Acquired Immune Deficiency Syndrome (A.I.D.S.)," *Journal of the American Institute of Homeopathy*, 80 (March 1987): 8–14.

45. Singh and Gupa, "Antiviral Efficacy."

46. R. G. Gibson et al., "Homoeopathic Therapy in Rheumatoid Arthritis: Evaluation by Double-Blind Clinical Therapeutic Trial," *British Journal of Clinical Pharmacology*, 9 (1980): 453–459.

See Appendix for updated information on homeopathy and AIDS

8

Allergic Conditions: Beyond Symptomatic Relief

The word *allergy* did not exist in Shakespeare's time or even just a century ago. And yet, medical statistics indicate that one in seven Americans had an allergy in 1950, as many as one in five had an allergy in 1970, and approximately 75 million Americans, or one in three, had an allergy in 1985.[1]

Allergy is a catchall word for a wide variety of reactions to substances that the body determines to be foreign. In a strict medical sense, the term refers to conditions that occur when the body's immune system is triggered and then overreacts to specific substances in the environment. These substances may be foods, animal hairs, house dust, pollens or other plant materials, molds, medicines, or chemicals.

The ability of the immune system to identify individual substances and to react to them is crucial for the body's protection. But overreaction to them leads to a variety of uncomfortable and sometimes dangerous symptoms. The most common include runny nose, sneezing, respiratory symptoms, watery eyes, headache, digestive symptoms, and skin symptoms. There are also various idiosyncratic symptoms that may occur.

Some people think of allergies as a single diagnostic category, but there are many different disease conditions that are allergic reactions. Hay fever is considered an allergic response to pollen. Asthma, hives, and eczema are also considered allergic conditions, though they can be triggered by psychological factors as well as by allergens.

Although it may be too late for most of us, perhaps the best way to prevent any of these allergic conditions is by being breast-fed during infancy. Bottle-fed babies are many times more suscep-tible to getting allergies than those who are breast-fed.[2] Mother's milk has important antibodies and other immunological factors that not only help to protect the infant but also help to develop the infant's immune system later in life.

The reason that respiratory and digestive symptoms are the most common reaction to allergens is that they both have a par-ticularly large number of "mast cells." Mast cells have histamine and various other chemicals locked inside, which are released when a person is exposed to allergens. Histamine dilates capillaries, which then increase the blood supply to peripheral parts of the body in defense against the invading allergen. Histamine also con-stricts the respiratory bronchioles, tubes that help the body to cough and expel the allergen. Finally, histamine causes increased gastric secretion in the body's effort to digest the allergen. Despite these various efforts by the body to try to protect and heal itself, the body is not always strong enough to effect a cure, and it some-times is so sick that it overreacts to substances that a healthy body can deal with effectively and without creating symptoms.

Conventional Medical Treatment for Allergies

The first step in the conventional medical treatment of allergic reactions is the use of antihistamines. These drugs, however, are considered ineffective in curing allergic reactions and at best only temporarily relieve some symptoms. This ineffectiveness is predic-table, since antihistamines do not treat the reason the mast cells are secreting histamine; instead, they suppress the body's reac-tion to an allergen and thereby only treat the symptoms of the problem, not the underlying disease. Also, recent research has recognized that the mast cells release other chemicals, including *leukotienes,* which cause inflammation and irritation. Although modern science is doing what it can to create drugs that have an anti-leukotienic effect, such drugs, like antihistamines, will inevitably only treat symptoms, not the disease. Because of this, anti-leukotienic drugs will have their side effects, too.

If antihistamines are ineffective or cause too much drowsiness or other symptoms, conventional physicians generally recommend steroid nasal spray. Steroidal (cortisone-like) drugs have a strong anti-inflammatory effect on the body and are particularly good at reducing swelling. When taken orally, these powerful drugs cause various serious symptoms, usually considerably worse than the simple allergic symptoms. Researchers have found that the steroid nasal sprays do not seem to cause these more serious symptoms. However, one must be suspicious of premature claims about their effectiveness or their limited side effects. These sprays have only recently been utilized. Their long-term effects are unknown, and since their action is only symptomatic, it is generally expected that allergic sufferers will need to use them over long periods of time.

The most recent development in the treatment of allergies is the use of laser surgery to vaporize mucus-forming nasal tissue. This radical treatment is symptomatic at best, and one must wonder if surgeons will at some point consider cutting off the nose of allergy sufferers.

People often use decongestants to treat allergies. Although these drugs initially reduce congestion, they produce a "rebound" effect in which the congestion gets worse than it was previously. These drugs, like too many conventional medications, simply suppress the body's efforts to deal with a stress, and they inevitably create more serious problems than they solve.

The next strategy in conventional medicine for the treatment of allergies is desensitization shots (often simply called "allergy shots"). This treatment, too, has its severe limitations, even according to the most respected medical authorities. Joe Graedon, author of *The People's Pharmacy*, notes that doctors do not even know how much of a dose the patient is getting when given an allergy shot. Ragweed pollen, grass pollen, and certain molds may have a *thousandfold* difference in strength, even when the manufacturer claims similar dosage.[3]

Desensitization shots are, by homeopathic standards, the least objectionable conventional treatment for allergies. The symptoms are not directly suppressed, and no strong doses of drugs are used. Because allergy shots are based on one of the basic principles of homeopathy, it can be conjectured that their partial success is due to their strengthening of the body's ability to deal with allergens more effectively. However, allergy shots are injected into the body in a way that the body is not commonly exposed to the allergens, and their efficacy may be reduced because of this mode of entry.

Although desensitization to bee stings and other insect venoms is generally effective, scientific studies on the effectiveness of desensitization to pollen, molds, house dust, and animal danders are generally inconclusive or lacking.[4]

The treatment of asthma is, as they say, a different ball game. This is not because conventional medications are particularly effective in curing this condition (they are not); rather, it is primarily because this condition is frightening and potentially fatal, and asthma medication that can effectively suppress symptoms is sometimes necessary.

In the past, the most common drug used to treat asthma symptoms was ephedrine, because it relaxes muscle spasms that constrict air passageways. Ephedrine, however, creates a host of side effects that make its use less valuable, especially for the long term or by those with hypertension, heart disease, thyroid disease, or prostate problems. It is sometimes prescribed with a barbiturate in order to limit its side effects, though this new combination drug creates its own set of symptoms.

Asthma patients are often given theophylline. This drug, which is chemically related to the caffeine in coffee, is temporarily helpful, but it, too, creates various side effects. It is ironic to note that homeopaths occasionally use microdoses of coffee to treat asthmatics, since coffee has been found to cause respiratory symptoms resembling asthma.

Another "coincidence" is that physicians sometimes prescribe ipratropium bromide, a drug related to atropine, for asthma. Atropine is a chief ingredient of *Belladonna,* another common homeopathic medicine given to asthmatics who have symptoms similar to those it has been found to cause. (See a homeopathic materia medica for details.)

In serious asthmatic attacks, physicians utilize steroids. These truly are graverobbers, often effectively reducing the life-threatening symptoms of asthma. Despite their essential value, however, steroids do not cure asthma, and the side effects from their long-term use are so severe that even the American Academy of Allergy does not condone their use except in life-threatening situations.[5]

Inhalers are helpful when used correctly for the less severe symptoms of asthma, and they generally have less severe side effects than other medications. Research has shown, however, that up to 77 percent of patients utilizing inhalers use them improperly, which significantly reduces the value of the drug.[6] People also tend to overuse the inhalers, creating both psychological and physiological dependence. Even those asthmatics who use the inhalers properly and in moderation find that the inhalers dry lung secretions, making it difficult for asthmatics to clear their chest and throat from mucus that is clogging their breathing passageway.

If all this sounds discouraging, it is even more distressing to note that asthmatics are often drug-sensitive. They are more apt than others to experience side effects from drugs, and therefore they are often prescribed additional drugs to deal with the side effects, which sometimes reduces the action of the asthma medication and creates a new set of side effects.

New drugs and procedures continue to be tested for the treatment of allergies and asthma. Some physicians predict that the future of allergy treatment lies in bone marrow transplants. Others say that "brain repair," in which new brain cells are actually grafted into the brain, is the wave of the future. And still others recommend new and more powerful drugs.[7] Some of these drugs and treatments initially may seem to have good effects on symptoms and few side effects. However, it is predictable that these drugs, too, will not be found to be effective and that the side effects from their long-term use will not warrant their prescription. This discouraging pattern of conventional drug use will continue until physicians and researchers develop a different understanding of allergies and of disease in general. Homeopathy offers an alternative.

The Homeopathic Treatment of Allergies

The homeopathic approach to treating allergies is, once again, based on the understanding that symptoms are the body's effort to correct an imbalance in the system. Rather than controlling or suppressing the symptoms, the homeopath prescribes a micro-dose of an individually chosen substance that has the capacity to create symptoms similar to those the allergic person is experiencing.

It should also be noted that there are some homeopathic medicines for acute allergy attacks and other homeopathic medicines for the underlying chronically ill state that gives rise to recurrent allergy symptoms. Whereas the acute medicine may be effective in reducing the allergy symptoms, it generally does not prevent these symptoms in the future. The medicine for the chronic state, in contrast, has the capacity to reduce the frequency or intensity of the allergy symptoms and can cure a person with allergy symptoms.

One of the common medicines given to people suffering from an acute allergy is *Allium cepa*, the onion. As is generally known, when cutting an onion one experiences a runny nose and tearing eyes, two common allergy symptoms. More specifically, *Allium cepa* causes a burning nasal discharge that irritates the nostrils and upper lip. It also causes redness and burning of the eyes, though the tears themselves do not irritate the eyelids or the cheeks. People with symptoms that require homeopathic doses of *Allium cepa* often think that the tissue paper they are using to wipe their noses is too rough, when, in fact, the tissue paper is as soft as it always is; the problem is that the nasal discharge has irritated the nostrils and made them more sensitive to touch. Like the symptoms that the onion creates when one is exposed to its juices, the symptoms of people who need this medicine are a nose and eye discharge that tends to be worse in warm rooms, indoors, and in the evening, and improved in open air. If these people suffer from frequent sneezing, they also find relief in the open air.

In contrast, people with acute allergy symptoms who need *Euphrasia* (eyebright) have a nonirritating, watery nasal discharge and copious burning tears (*Allium cepa* causes a burning nasal discharge and nonburning tears). People who need *Euphrasia* feel worse in the open air, in the morning, and while lying down. They may have a loose cough, though it is not usually deep or severe. The cough is worse during the day and may only occur during the daytime. It is relieved at night by eating and by lying down, though lying down makes the nasal symptoms worse.

The treatment of chronic allergies, like the treatment of any chronic symptoms, requires the care of a professional homeopath. Although there are only a dozen or so homeopathic medicines commonly given for acute allergy symptoms, there are several hundred medicines that homeopaths must consider when treating chronic allergies.

Besides the successes that homeopaths report from their clinical practice, there has also been some good research providing evidence of the value of the homeopathic medicines in reducing allergic responses. Some French researchers have found that *Apis* (crushed bee) and *Histamine* in homeopathic microdoses have a statistically significant effect on reducing the allergic response.[8]

Apis is a common homeopathic medicine for various allergic symptoms, since the symptoms it causes resemble an allergic condition. *Apis*, for instance, is one of the common medicines given to people with hives. As is generally known, bee venom causes a burning, stinging pain that is relieved by ice or cold applications and aggravated by heat or warm applications or by simple covering. If a person with hives has his condition aggravated by direct heat, warm applications, or from the body becoming heated from exertion, *Apis* may be the medicine of choice. It is particularly indicated when the hives are triggered by eating shellfish or when there is swelling around the eyes.

Another medicine given for hives is *Urtica urens*, the stinging nettle. Those people who live in the temperate climates where it grows know that simply touching the nettle's stem or stalk causes a hivelike reaction. As with *Apis*, the hives are made worse by warmth or exercise. People who need *Urtica urens*, however, get noticeable relief when lying down, but they are aggravated again upon getting up. They have an urge to rub the hives constantly, but this can exacerbate the condition. The hives can be triggered after eating pork or pastries.

Hay fever is another condition for which homeopathy has been shown to offer effective treatment. In a double-blind clinical study done by representatives of the Glasgow Homeopathic Hospital in collaboration with researchers from the University of Glasgow, it was found that homeopathy was successful in significantly diminishing the symptoms of hay fever. The study of 144 patients with hay fever, which was published in the prestigious medical journal *Lancet*, showed that those given a homeopathic dose of mixed pollen medicine (a mixture of twelve different species of grass pollens given in a potency of 30c*) had six times as much improvement as did those who were given a placebo. In the study, subjects were allowed to take a conventional drug that temporarily diminished symptoms if they felt they needed this relief. Those patients who were given the homeopathic medicine required this drug half as often as those people given the placebo.[9]

Despite the success of using this medicine or several other homeopathic medicines for acute hay fever symptoms, homeopaths generally assume that hay fever is a sign of an underlying chronic weakness that requires professional homeopathic care. Even if microdoses effectively reduce or eliminate hay fever symptoms, it is still recommended that one see a homeopath. And if a homeopathic medicine alone does not work for a person, or if it only relieves hay fever temporarily, it is strongly recommended that he or she seek professional homeopathic care.

The homeopathic treatment of asthma, like the homeopathic treatment of any chronic or serious condition, definitely requires professional care. Such care is often particularly problematic because the curative process is not always immediate, and in the meantime asthmatic attacks may occur that require medical intervention with conventional drugs. These drugs, though useful in dealing with an acute asthma attack, may inhibit the action of the homeopathic medicine and thereby delay cure of the condition, contributing to a nonproductive cycle of aggravation and

---

*30c is a dose that has been diluted at the ratio of one part medicine to 100 parts distilled water and then shaken vigorously; this process is repeated thirty times.

suppression.

Homeopathic medicines may not be able to effect a cure with every individual, but homeopaths commonly find that microdoses can strengthen physiological defenses to reduce the frequency and severity of asthma. Homeopaths and their patients can often cite cases in which there was complete cure of asthma, but it is as yet uncertain how frequently the medicines act in this thorough a fashion.

The homeopathic treatment of asthma generally involves constitutional care, which involves the strict individualization of medicines based on the totality of the person's symptoms, past and present. Most commonly, a single medicine is not enough to effect a cure, and a series of medicines over a period of several months or years are needed.

The homeopathic treatment of eczema provides a classic example of the difference between conventional and homeopathic care. Conventional treatment of eczema generally involves the use of steroid creams or, in severe cases, of oral cortisone in order to control the allergic response. Homeopaths do not think of eczema as a skin condition, but assume that the epidermal symptoms represent an underlying disease process. Homeopathic treatment is then based on the individual prescription of a substance that has the capacity to cause, when given in overdose, dermal, digestive, respiratory, eliminatory, psychological, and various other symptoms similar to those the person experiences.

Eczema is certainly an irritating condition, but from the homeopathic point of view this skin problem represents a superficial rather than a deep disease. Hering's Law of Cure, which was discussed in detail in Chapter 1, affirms the homeopathic view that skin symptoms generally are the least threatening to survival of the organism. Although skin symptoms still represent an illness, control or suppression of these symptoms delay cure and increase the possibility of more serious side effects.

Certain foods may be a triggering factor in eczema. Since food allergies are of growing concern, it is worthwhile to provide the homeopathic perspective and treatment of such conditions.

The Homeopathic
Treatment of Food Allergies

It is easy to be confused about food allergies. Many of us notice
that certain foods do not "agree" with us, but it is uncertain if
we are actually allergic to them or if our symptoms are primarily
psychosomatic. Since some people with food allergies do not react
to the food immediately after eating it but several hours or even
days later, it is difficult to determine if our ill feeling is the result
of something we ate or some other factor. Some natural healers
or diet experts also diagnose people as having several food allergies,
even when the person seems relatively well and without significant symptoms. The individual is told that these "allergies" are
a latent problem that will cause symptoms at some point in the
future unless something is done.

It should be noted that conventional tests for allergies are
notoriously inaccurate, and the various alternative testing methods
(clinical ecology, muscle-testing, cytotoxic testing, iridology, and
psychic diagnosis) have not yet been proven to be any better.

Once a person is "diagnosed" as allergic to a specific food,
it is generally recommended that he or she avoid that particular
food.* From a homeopathic point of view, this may reduce some
of the person's symptoms, but it certainly does not cure the person. Simply avoiding a stress does not strengthen an organism.

The homeopathic approach is to take a detailed case history
of the person's physical and psychological symptoms. In this history, the homeopath always asks the person what foods seem to
cause symptoms. The homeopath also asks what foods the person
craves or dislikes. This information helps the homeopath to find

---

*It is interesting to note that physicians who specialize in clinical
ecology, which is a sophisticated though not consistently accurate method
of testing for allergies, seek to reduce a food allergy by giving small,
gradually increasing doses of food to which the person is allergic. Although this is not the classical homeopathic approach, it does have
homeopathic elements.

a homeopathic medicine that is uniquely matched to the total psycho-physical metabolic state of the sick person, not just the one allergic reaction.

Homeopathy is sometimes rapid in curing food allergies, though more often it takes time. In the process of cure, here are some helpful guidelines that may help the reader to feel less confused about food allergies and to make decisions about them.

1. Human beings are physically capable of eating almost any type of vegetable or animal tissue except woody cellulose and lignin. Some types of foods are not easily digested, and these should simply not be eaten in quantity. There are undoubtedly optimum ranges for the amount of each type of food that should be included in one's diet, but people in various cultures have thrived and lived to old age on different sorts of diets.

2. Few of us suffer from food allergies or other significant adverse reactions to foods. A person who pays attention to how he or she feels and is healthy in general, including after eating, can be assumed to be free of such problems.

3. Because each person is a unique individual, he or she will respond uniquely to foods. Most of us can become aware of what foods "agree" with us and what foods leave us feeling queasy or drowsy or some other way that just does not feel right. It makes sense to choose the staples of one's diet from the former group and to not eat too much of the latter.

4. Sometimes people react to foods only on rare occasions. This may be because of a specific combination of foods that is difficult to digest. In such cases—if this combination of foods frequently causes some difficulty—one might avoid these foods together. At other times, a hypersensitivity to an individual food may only be temporary or seasonal. And at still other times, the symptoms may not be related to the food at all but to the person's psychological state at the time. Such temporary hypersensitivities should not be thought of as allergies, and one should not avoid a food simply because one has occasionally had problems with it.

5. Significant adverse reactions to food do occur and can cause a wide variety of symptoms in some individuals. Children are

particularly prone to food allergies. Because of the great variability of symptoms, and because the symptoms sometimes do not manifest themselves until hours or even days after the food is ingested, the diagnosis of food allergies is frequently not considered when it should be.

6. A person can sometimes diagnose food allergies on his own without the supervision of a health professional. The elimination diet is a method whereby one totally drops selected foods from his diet for a period of three or four weeks. Usually, the offending food is one that is eaten regularly and one for which the person may have a craving. The most common allergic foods are milk, eggs, chocolate, corn, wheat, citrus fruits, beans and peas, tomatoes, nuts, fish, preservatives, and colas. After avoiding potential offending foods for three or four weeks, the person eats a fairly large portion of a single food. He or she then makes note of what symptoms, if any, occur.*

Diagnosing what food allergies one has may be beneficial in some ways, though simply avoiding certain foods does not cure the underlying weakness that created the problem in the first place. Homeopathic medicines, on the other hand, offer a real potential for cure from food allergies. The medicines strengthen the overall functioning of the organism and reestablish healthy digestion, assimilation, and elimination of foods.

Whether one has hay fever, asthma, eczema, or any other allergic response, the homeopath assumes that the "problem" is not the specific substance to which the person is reacting. The problem is the person's overreactive body that is hypersensitive to it. Homeopathy is a sophisticated method that not only can reduce the frequency and severity of allergy symptoms but also can increase a person's overall level of health. Although more research certainly needs to be done on the homeopathic treatment of allergies, it is worthwhile to try homeopathy. The only thing you have

---

*More detail about the elimination diet method can be obtained by reading Alan Scott Levin and Merla Zellerbach, *The Type 1/Type 2 Allergy Relief Program* (Los Angeles: J. P. Tarcher, 1983); or Natalie Golas and Frances Golos Golbitz, *Coping with Your Allergies* (New York: Fireside, 1986).

to lose is your sniffles, your digestive problems, and your headaches.

Notes

1. Alan Scott Levin and Merla Zellerbach, *The Type 1/Type 2 Allergy Relief Program* (Los Angeles, J. P. Tarcher, 1983), p. 25.

2. Robert Mendelsohn, *How to Raise a Healthy Child . . . In Spite of Your Doctor* (Chicago: Contemporary Books, 1984), p. 194.

3. Joe Graedon, *The People's Pharmacy* (New York: St. Martin's Press, 1985), pp. 307–308.

4. Philip S. Norman, "An Overview of Immunotherapy: Implications for the Future," *Journal of Allergy and Clinical Immunology*, 65 (1980): 87–96.

5. Earl B. Brown, "Reply to Corticosteroid Therapy in Asthma," *Journal of Allergy*, 41 (1968): 60.

6. D. Appel, "Faulty Use of Canister Nebulizers for Asthma," *Journal of Family Practice*, 14 (1982): 1135–39.

7. Levin and Zellerbach, *Type 1/Type 2*, pp. 178–181.

8. Jean Boiron, Jacky Abecassis, and Philippe Belon, eds., "The Effects of Hahnemannian Potencies of 7c *Histaminum* and 7c *Apis Mellifica* upon Basophil Degranulation in Allergic Patients," in *Aspects of Research in Homeopathy* (Lyon: Boiron, 1983), pp. 61–67.

9. David Taylor Reilly, Morag A. Taylor, Charles McSharry, and Tom Aitchison, "Is Homoeopathy a Placebo Response? Controlled Trial of Homoeopathic Potency, with Pollen in Hayfever as Model," *Lancet*, 8512 (October 18, 1986): 881–886.

9

The Treatment of Chronic Disease: The Homeopathic Alternative

Every couple of months, reports in newspapers and on television announce success in treating yet another health problem. Despite these advances, as Lewis Thomas, the head of the famed Sloan-Kettering Institute, has admitted, "the truth is that there are not nearly as many [advances] as the public has been led to believe."[1]

If the various media reports on medical advances were true, then we certainly would have been able to cure nearly every disease by now. Sadly, this is not the case. The media have tended to report the initial successes of medical procedures. Later, when these procedures are tested more extensively, they are usually found to be either not as effective as previously considered or more harmful than beneficial. These reports, however, are not "hot news."

The conventional medical treatment for cancer is a classic example of this phenomenon. Over the past several decades, the National Cancer Institute and several other cancer research centers have asserted that victory over cancer is just around the corner—if only the government and the public would continue to give them vast sums of money. Cancer researchers have continually reported on their "impressive" progress, but have manipulated statistics in a questionably ethical manner. A recent comprehensive review of cancer research in the *New England Journal of Medicine* announced that "we are losing the war against cancer."[2] This report showed that modern medical treatment for cancer is not reducing the number of people suffering from this disease nor is it adequately increasing the five-year cancer survival rate.

The National Cancer Institute estimates that more than 200,000 patients receive chemotherapy in the United States each year. A recent article in the *Scientific American* expressed serious concern about this large number, stating: "For a dangerous and technologically exacting form of treatment, these are disturbing figures, particularly since the benefit for most categories of patients has yet to be established. Furthermore, the number of patients who are being cured can hardly amount to more than a few percent of those who are treated."[3] But despite this dismal analysis of cancer treatment, the general public has been given a very different message from the press. As Dr. D. S. Greenberg observed in the *New England Journal of Medicine,* "the lay press is unduly gullible in reporting 'progress' in cancer treatment."[4]

The possibility of near victory over cancer is reminiscent of similar claims by American military generals of certain victory in Vietnam if only the government would increase its funding. Journalist Peter Barry Chowka has extended this analogy further by noting that the cancer patient today undergoes a "Vietnamization of the body." He is hit with surgical strikes, burned, and poisoned with toxic chemicals, while in most cases the elusive enemy melts away, soon to surface in more deadly forms elsewhere. The doctors destroy his body in order to save it.[5]

Whereas modern medicine claims great success in treating a wide range of acute diseases and medical emergencies, it is generally acknowledged that modern medicine has little to offer most people with chronic illnesses. The treatments are primarily palliative, rarely curative.

It is no accident, then, that Americans consume over 20,000 tons of aspirin per year—or 225 tablets each. Although aspirin may relieve our pain temporarily, it does nothing to deal with the underlying processes that create the pain in the first place.

It is no accident that over 20 percent of patients discharged from hospitals are rehospitalized within two months, generally for the *same* illness for which they were originally hospitalized.[6] Palliation and suppression of symptoms not only do not work but can cause serious symptoms, and potentially death.

It is no accident that conventional drugs cause serious side effects. A recent article published in the *Journal of the American Medical Association* reported that the Food and Drug Administration receives thousands of reports each year about adverse reactions to drugs. In 1984 the FDA received 30,000 such reports, and in 1985 there were almost 40,000 reports.[7]

It is no accident that the vast majority of drugs listed in the *Physicians' Desk Reference* are not listed in this book only ten years later. Conventional doctors call this "progress." It generally means that new, questionably effective drugs have replaced the old, ineffective drugs, which will themselves be replaced soon.

Conventional drugs may be helpful in relieving pain, but, sadly enough, these drugs rarely cure and too often they do more harm than good.

To make matters worse, chronic disease is on the rise. Whereas significant numbers of people died of acute infectious disease at the turn of the century, today significant numbers of people die of chronic disease. Chronic disease is not increasing simply because we are living longer, for there is now evidence that chronic disease is increasing for people at younger and younger ages.

According to the National Center for Health Statistics, the percentage of persons under seventeen years of age who are limited in activity due to chronic conditions increased by 86 percent from 1967 to 1979.[8] This limitation in activity increased by 21 percent for people between the ages of seventeen and forty-four.[9] The rate of heart disease in the United States is the highest in the world; and although this condition has diminished greatly over the past decade, hypertension for people under the age of forty-five has increased significantly when compared to the late 1960s.

There are many reasons for the increase in chronic disease. One contributing factor is that conventional medicine offers little in terms of curative treatment, and many of its therapies actually foster the development of serious health problems. One study published in the *New England Journal of Medicine* in 1981 showed that 36 percent of patients in a respected university's hospital were admitted for an iatrogenic (doctor-induced) illness.[10]

The conventional medical treatment for heart disease provides an excellent example of questionably effective medical care. Although the rate of heart disease has decreased in the past decade, its incidence was so high in the 1970s that it is difficult to imagine it doing anything *but* decreasing. There are still approximately 600,000 deaths from heart disease in the United States every year, which alone is about half the number of all reported births.

Almost 90 percent of Americans with heart disease have coronary artery disease, a condition in which the heart's arteries are partially blocked, causing decreased oxygen to the heart. *Propranolol* (Inderal) is one of the common medicines for coronary disease because it reduces the heart's need for oxygen by reducing its ability to pump blood. As it does this, however, it also reduces the heart's ability to respond to exercise. And for some people, it can aggravate lung disease or cause heart failure, fatigue, depression, and impotence.

Physicians use various medications to lower blood pressure, and it is generally expected that people will need to stay on these drugs at least as long as their blood pressure remains high—which is usually the remainder of their lives, since nothing is actually done to deal with the underlying reasons for the high blood pressure. Using these medications in old age, however, carries additional health risks. As people age, the flow of blood to their brains is reduced. A further reduction as the result of medication can exacerbate various physical or mental conditions.[11]

Coronary bypass surgery is a process of removing a vein from a patient's leg and splicing it to a coronary artery as a way of providing a detour for blood to pass around a blocked artery. Although there has been a decrease in heart disease, the amount of bypass surgeries has increased astronomically. In 1977 there were 50,000 bypass surgeries, and in 1986 there were over 200,000 of them. It should be noted that although these surgeries have been found to diminish pain, there is insufficient evidence that they enable people to live longer.

Because people with coronary disease have various emotional symptoms that accompany their physical symptoms, physicians often prescribe valium or librium to reduce anxiety. They prescribe other drugs to reduce platelet clumping in order to decrease further clotting of the arteries, and still other drugs to reduce coronary artery spasms.

These drugs and surgical procedures are classical examples of treating symptoms rather than the underlying disease. Since a person's body develops its symptoms over several years or even decades, altering the heart's intricate physiological processes with strong drugs can wreak havoc. By reducing one's blood pressure without dealing with the various reasons the body has developed this condition, one inevitably creates side effects that are not simply "side" effects but direct effects of drug treatment.

These drugs and surgical procedures can be lifesaving, but there is growing evidence of safer methods of reducing the life-threatening nature of heart disease. Dr. I. Hjermann and colleagues reported in *Lancet* that in a study of 1,200 men between the ages of forty and forty-nine who were at high risk of coronary heart disease, there was a 47 percent lower rate of heart attacks and sudden cardiac deaths after the men reduced their cigarette smoking and the amount of animal products consumed.[12]

Dr. Julian Whitaker, author of *Reversing Heart Disease*, estimates that as many as 80 percent of coronary bypass surgeries would be unnecessary if doctors would inform their patients of less radical treatment options, such as a sensible diet and exercise program.[13]

Homeopathic medicine offers a safe option to persons with heart disease and other chronic illnesses. In order to understand what homeopaths have to offer, it is necessary to understand first what homeopaths think about the nature of chronic disease.

The Homeopaths'
Understanding of Chronic Disease

The vast majority of the survivors of Hiroshima and Nagasaki died of leukemia, sometimes five, ten, fifteen, or even twenty years later. The fact that they survived without initial symptoms does not mean that they were completely healthy prior to the diagnosis of leukemia.

Leukemia, like many other kinds of cancer, does not seem to have forewarning symptoms; and by the time it can be diagnosed, it is often difficult to treat successfully. Since cancer usually takes many years or perhaps decades to develop, its effects on the body prior to diagnosis can be very subtle.

Homeopathic medicine provides a system of selecting medicines according to the totality of subtle and overt symptoms of the body and mind. Without necessarily needing to know why a person has constipation, flatulence after eating certain foods, hypersensitivity to cold, low energy upon waking, depression when alone, or any other idiosyncratic symptom, homeopaths prescribe a microdose of a medicine that has the capacity to create a similar set of subtle or overt symptoms. For whatever reason the body creates its symptoms, the correct homeopathic medicine augments the body's ability to defend or heal itself.

Homeopaths believe that symptoms are manifestations of the defenses of the organism attempting to heal itself. At the very first level of defense, an *eliminative process* is initiated as the organic systems of the body respond to stress or infection by increasing their defensive function, often subtly and without the conscious awareness of the individual. The gastrointestinal, respiratory, circulatory, lymphatic, neuroendocrine, and/or genitourinary systems are stimulated in a concerted effort to reestablish homeostasis.

Once this defensive response reaches a certain level, the person actually begins to feel the reactions of his or her body and experiences *sensory changes*. The philosopher Descartes described the purpose of this intrinsic survival mechanism well: "The great engineer of the universe has made man as perfectly as he could make him, and he could not have invented a better device for his maintenance than to provide him with a sense of pain."

The third level of defense is *functional*. The body is not as able or as efficient in certain functions. The organic systems begin to suffer, sometimes overfunctioning in efforts to heal the organism, and sometimes underfunctioning as the result of exhaustion or of interference from other organic systems. The problems that the body has as it tries to eliminate the debris of metabolism may create local or general symptoms. The intercellular space (the cells' environment) will not enable the cells to nurture themselves; and if the eliminative processes are not functioning properly, *functional disturbances* ensue. A person with indigestion is less able to digest additional food efficiently and may experience nausea, vomiting, or diarrhea. A person with respiratory congestion is less able to oxygenate his cells, with the result that he gets out of breath easily.

If the stress or infection that is creating the defense reaction is particularly strong or persistent, if the person's body is weakened for whatever reason, or if the body's efforts to defend itself are suppressed (which is too often the case with the use of conventional medicines), the body is not always able to heal itself. The sensory and functional symptoms then become *chronic*.

Chronic symptoms stress the body, weaken its ability to deal with new stresses or infections, and decrease its efficient functioning. In efforts to deal with and adapt to chronic symptoms, the body draws on various creative means to defend and heal itself. These efforts lead to *pathological and structural tissue change.*

An example of the disease process evolving from an initial stress to ultimate pathological tissue change can be seen in the case of constipation. At first, there may be slight, perhaps even unnoticeable, changes in bowel function. The sensory changes may then become more obvious, with the person having an uncomfortable feeling in the abdomen and increased difficulty in eliminating stools. Next, functional changes may develop: the person may have less energy and may experience indigestion as well as various other bodily and psychological symptoms. The chronic functional disturbances may then lead to pathological tissue changes. At first, hemorrhoids may be experienced, diverticulosis (a protusion in the large intestine resulting from weakness in the muscular layer of the bowel) may be the second stage of tissue change, and cancer of the colon may be the third stage.*

The body continually tries to defend and heal itself in each stage of disease, based on its capabilities at the time. When something is done for the body (for example, giving hormones to a person who secretes too few; giving laxatives to a person who is constipated; or giving antihistamines to a person to dry up his mucous membranes), the body is sometimes habituated away from developing the correct healing process on its own. In fact, these efforts to do something *for* the body tend primarily to suppress the body's

---

*For more information on the various stages of disease, see Hans-Heinrich Reckeweg, *Homotoxicology* (Albuquerque: Menaco, 1980).

ability to act independently, often creating an addiction, causing a rebound effect in which the symptoms are experienced with greater intensity, and producing more severe disease.

Homeopaths conjecture that one major reason there is more chronic disease today is precisely *because* of the suppressive nature of conventional medical therapies.

Although this suppressive treatment may contribute to chronic disease, it is certainly not the only cause. Hahnemann was ahead of his time as an environmentalist as well as a physician. He acknowledged that toxic exposure to certain minerals and chemicals in the environment and workplace can lead to disease, and he asserted that unless the "obstacle to cure" is dealt with in such cases, cure will be incomplete.

Hahnemann and most homeopaths since him have also acknowledged an hereditary influence on chronic disease. Hahnemann referred to the "miasmatic" state as the underlying susceptibility primarily responsible for the various acute and chronic illnesses that people experience. He theorized three primary "miasms." The first miasm is called "psora," the meaning of which has been debated since Hahnemann first named it. Basically, it refers to an underlying deficiency and susceptibility to disease. Referred to as the "mother of chronic disease," psora is the primary weakened state that allows a susceptibility to a host of chronic diseases. The other two miasms were related to the venereal diseases: syphilis and gonorrhea. Hahnemann asserted that the ineffectual, usually suppressive, treatment of syphilis and gonorrhea leads to a chronic miasm that not only can create various serious chronic disease states but can be genetically passed on to one's children or grandchildren.

Not every homeopath adopted Hahnemann's theory of miasms, and most conventional physicians dismissed it as preposterous. Actually, Hahnemann's miasmatic theory makes new sense in the context of the present understanding of genetics and physiology. First of all, it is common knowledge that prior to the 1940s conventional physicians used various mercury mixtures to treat people with syphilis. Although this treatment sometimes diminished the chancre, it often did not cure the person's syphilis. The person did not die immediately, but continued to live for several years, usually with serious neurological and skeletal abnormalities prior to death. Before dying, it is quite possible that this person made love with another, leading to the birth of a baby. This baby may not necessarily have syphilis as a disease, but might experience the hereditary effects of his father's or mother's syphilis.

It is quite possible that a similar type of process could have occurred if a father, mother, or distant relative had gonorrhea that was not successfully treated and that eventually was passed down to the children.

And it is quite possible that there may be other diseases within our families that were not successfully treated in the past and that affect our health today. It is now known that the DNA of certain viruses can be incorporated into the genetic material of cells and thus be passed on to future generations. We may, in fact, be adding new miasms to our lineage by the ineffective, suppressive treatment of many of today's illnesses.

It should be noted that the miasms do not always lead to specific diseases but rather to types of constitutional conditions that affect the way a person experiences diseases. For instance, homeopaths have found that people with the gonorrheal miasm tend to manifest symptoms of overgrowth of tissue (enlarged organs, tumors, warts, fibrous growths or cysts, excess weight), accumulation of mucus, and disturbances of the pelvic and sexual organs.* These people's symptoms tend to be improved after they experience a discharge of some sort and to worsen if discharges are suppressed. Persons with this miasm also experience aggravation of symptoms during cold, wet weather. They may be restless (physically and mentally), cross, irritable, absentminded, selfish, and mischievous.

In contrast, individuals with the syphilitic miasm tend to manifest ulcerations of various sorts (in the stomach or duodenum, or in mucous membranes), deformities of the bones and tissues (protuding forehead, big lips, malformed nails, balding), destruction of tissue leading to hemorrhaging and blood disorders, and varicose veins. These people usually experience aggravation of

---

*In the homeopathic literature, the gonorrhea miasm is called the "sycotic miasm." "Sycotic" means figwart, referring to growth of tissue.

symptoms at night and after sweating. Unlike those with the gonorrheal miasm, those with the syphilitic miasm do not feel better after discharges. They are mentally dull, heavy, stupid, stubborn, and sullen. They are prone to alcoholism and violence, and in extreme cases can develop a desire to destroy things, kill others, or commit suicide.

It should be noted that these descriptions are only simple generalizations of complex typologies. For more detail about these miasmatic types, see Hahnemann's *Chronic Diseases*, Roberts's *Art of Cure by Homoeopathy*, Kent's *Lectures on Homoeopathic Philosophy*, Allen's *Chronic Miasms*, or Ortega's *Notes on the Miasms*.[14]

Miasmatic theory puts chronic disease in an hereditary context. Treatment of chronic disease with homeopathy requires a much more extensive knowledge of homeopathy than the treatment of acute disease. Whereas homeopaths often encourage people to treat themselves for acute, nonserious diseases or injuries, there is general agreement among them that the treatment of chronic disease requires professional homeopathic care.

The implication of miasmatic theory is that acute symptoms are sometimes the result of the person's miasmatic state. If, for instance, a person treats himself or herself for an acute condition on a couple of occasions but the condition persists or returns, it can be assumed that a deeper-acting medicine, or what is sometimes called a "miasmatic medicine," is needed. Professional homeopathic care is once again indicated in such conditions.

In addition to using miasmatic theory to understand and treat chronic disease, knowledge of other basic homeopathic principles can also be helpful in aiding science to understand what factors may lead to certain diseased states. Alzheimer's disease is a case in point. A form of senile dementia, Alzheimer's disease has become the fourth leading cause of death among people sixty-five years old or older and presently afflicts over two million Americans. Autopsies of the brain cells of some, but not all, Alzheimer's patients have found increased concentrations of aluminum. Because physicians tend not to acknowledge factors that lead to disease except when these factors occur in *virtually every* case, the problems that aluminum creates have not been fully appreciated. One medical newsletter theorized that "the presence of aluminum could as easily be the result of the disease as its cause."[15]

Whatever the reason aluminum is found in the brains of certain people, it is advisable in general to avoid ingestion of it. Thus, it is recommended that people not use aluminum cookware or antacid pills (since these pills have aluminum in them).

The reason that homeopaths have discouraged the use of aluminum cookware for over one hundred years is that they know what effects it has in overdose. A British homeopath recently listed the primary symptoms of Alzheimer's disease and noted that *each* of these symptoms is an aspect of what aluminum causes in overdose.[16]

The present scientific attitude toward the connection between Alzheimer's disease and aluminum is reminiscent of the attitude just a couple of decades ago when it was not yet "fully proven" that smoking causes lung cancer. There may indeed be other factors that also lead to Alzheimer's disease, just as there are reasons other than smoking that lead to lung cancer. However, evidence presently suggests that aluminum is a primary factor in this condition, and that unless people stop their use of aluminum cookware and antacid pills, the Alzheimer epidemic will spread.

By investigating the various homeopathic materia medicas, we can learn an enormous amount about what various plants, minerals, animals, and chemicals cause in overdose. We can then discover why some people become ill. A veritable treasure house of information awaits us in these homeopathic texts.*

There is an old Chinese proverb that says: "If we do not change our direction, we are liable to end up where we are headed." It seems clear that our present approach to chronic disease is not working as well as doctors or patients would like. Rather than devoting more research and manpower to provide more people with this kind of care, we should consider changing our direction. It is time to consider homeopathic medicine.

---

*Only a small number of people become ill because of toxic exposure to a single substance. Still, by understanding why a small number of people get ill, it sometimes leads to greater understanding of the healing and diseasing process in general.

The Homeopathic Treatment
of Chronic Diseases

"Nature's ever open book, . . . come to us, page by page, word by word, and letter by letter, in the form of living human beings that are technically called patients," wrote Dr. J. Compton Burnett in *Diseases of the Veins.* In "A Country Doctor," a short story by Franz Kafka, one character criticizes a conventional doctor, noting: "To write prescriptions is easy, but to come to an understanding with people is hard." The homeopathic approach to understanding people is decidedly "hard." One must conduct a detailed interview of the various overt and subtle physical, emotional, and mental symptoms. One must elicit these symptoms without putting words into the patient's mouth. One must develop trust, use intuition and insight, and be mentally and emotionally clear enough to absorb and interpret this information. To come to an understanding with people is hard; yet the use of homeopathic medicines helps make this effort worth it.

Homeopathy developed its popularity in the 19th century thanks to its success in treating epidemic diseases. Today it is developing its reputation by providing effective health care for chronic diseases. Two centuries of clinical experience have demonstrated the effectiveness of homeopathy. There have also been some good double-blind studies that have confirmed the efficacy of homeopathic medicines in treating chronic disease. In 1980, the *British Journal of Clinical Pharmacology* published a double-blind study that showed the impressive effects of homeopathic medicines on people suffering from rheumatoid arthritis. Researchers found that 82 percent of those given homeopathic medicines experienced some type of benefit, while only 21 percent of those given a placebo experienced a similar degree of improvement.[17]

The fact that homeopathy offers effective and safe treatment for people with rheumatoid arthritis is of special significance. Rheumatoid arthritis is considered an autoimmune disease—that is, one in which the immune system begins attacking the body's own cells. The beneficial treatment of this form of arthritis suggests that homeopathic medicines influence the body's immune system. If this is true (as many homeopaths believe), the potential for homeopathic medicine in treating a wide variety of acute and chronic conditions is immense, since the immune system plays such a crucial role in the healing process.

There have been similar double-blind experiments on the homeopathic treatment of hay fever[18] and fibrositis (a rheumatic condition).[19] Both of these studies have shown that the health of people can be improved with the use of homeopathic medicines as compared with the health of those given a placebo.*

In addition to these scientific studies, the homeopathic literature is replete with case histories by physicians who have treated a panoply of chronic illnesses successfully. Although these case histories do not in themselves "prove" homeopathy, the fact that hundreds of thousands of physicians and tens of millions of patients have experienced beneficial results with the homeopathic medicines suggests that these may indeed have some value.

Homeopathic medicine, of course, cannot accomplish the impossible. It cannot heal people whose immune and defense systems have been severely compromised as the result of long-term use of suppressive medications. It cannot heal people whose pathology has developed into certain organic, structural diseases for which surgery is indicated. And it cannot heal people whose pathology is primarily the result of certain particularly stressful lifestyle or environmental factors from which they do not want to or are unable to extricate themselves.

Despite these predictable limitations, effective treatment with homeopathic medicines is possible for the vast numbers of people with chronic illness today. *Real* cure is possible with homeopathy. The medicines catalyze an overall healing response in the organism that creates a higher level of order and function. As the result of this increased integrity, not only do symptoms of chronic com-

---

*More research will indeed be helpful in informing health professionals and the general public about homeopathy's benefits. Consult the Resources section in Part III of this book for the addresses of organizations sponsoring new homeopathic research and providing education about previous research.

plaint become resolved, but people say that they feel noticeably better in general, physically and psychologically. It is quite common, in fact, for people to say that they have never felt better than after taking an individually prescribed homeopathic medicine. It is also quite common for people to be able to make important decisions dealing with their job, their family, their lover, or their life in general after taking a homeopathic medicine. And people occasionally describe having dreams and premonitions of personal significance after taking a homeopathic medicine.

Although surgery may be indicated for certain people, there are innumerable instances in which homeopathic medicines prevent its necessity, including cases of breast and ovarian cysts, uterine fibroids, enlarged thyroid, kidney stones, gallstones, chronically swollen tonsils or adenoids, and instances of recurrent vaginal bleeding for which a hysterectomy is too often the treatment of choice. Each of these and other potential surgical conditions requires individual assessment to determine if a homeopathic medicine can help. Since surgery is a radical form of treatment, more conservative methods such as homeopathic medicines play an invaluable role in providing good health care.

One of the most common sayings in homeopathy is that "there are no incurable diseases, only incurable people." By this, homeopaths mean that it is not the specific disease that limits the potential for healing but the strength of the person's defenses and the ability of the practitioner to find the correct remedy to stimulate those defenses.

Most people do not experience "a cure" after taking a single medicine. A large number may experience some significant progress toward health after taking a single medicine, but usually a series of individually prescribed medicines over several months— or, in some cases, over years—is needed for a deep healing process to take place.

For various reasons, known and unknown, it is particularly difficult to prescribe accurately for some people. If people have used conventional drugs for long periods of time, or if they are presently taking conventional medications, their real symptoms are masked by the actions of the drugs. It is difficult to withdraw some people, notably diabetics and epileptics, from their medications. Homeopaths have achieved some success in treating these people, but such patients are carefully monitored medically, and, if possible, their medications are slowly reduced. It is rare for homeopaths to be able to withdraw a diabetic completely from his or her insulin, though they are sometimes able to reduce the amount of insulin needed, and sometimes the homeopathic medicines seem to improve the person's overall health and prevent complications of the disease process. It is possible for homeopathy to work in tandem with drug replacement therapy.

It is also difficult to treat some people who are hypersensitive to certain substances in the environment and to many drugs. Homeopaths have noted that these people tend to be hypersensitive to homeopathic drugs, too. The homeopathic medicines sometimes help them profoundly, but oftentimes only seem to change the person's symptoms without really curing the person.

Finally, some people are difficult to cure for unknown reasons. It is not that these people are necessarily deeply ill; it is just that, for unknown reasons, the correct homeopathic medicine cannot be found. The person may have a chronic headache, or a persistent skin condition, or an irritating digestive problem. When possible, homeopaths refer these people to a fellow homeopath in the hope that another practitioner will be able to provide some new insight about the person in the search for the correct medicine. At other times, homeopaths, like other health professionals, will refer to other specialists, both conventional medical specialists and practitioners that specialize in natural therapies. It is important to reiterate that homeopaths are not "against" conventional therapies; rather, as physicians and healers, they simply prefer to try less invasive measures first.

A Case of Undiagnosed Chronic Abdominal Pain

At the age of nineteen, my sister Dyan began to experience a sharp, daily abdominal pain in her lower right side. Despite thorough examinations by five specialists and an exploratory surgery, no diagnosis could be made and no treatment was effective. Her condition persisted for two years.

Although I had an interest in homeopathy and other natural healing systems, my sister had no interest in these alternatives. Since our father is a pediatrician of the conventional school of medicine, she wanted to follow his advice, not mine.

Several months after her unsuccessful exploratory surgery, I asked her if she would like to try homeopathy. She said she was not interested. When I told her that she had nothing to lose, that homeopathic medicines do not have any side effects, and that she could concurrently do whatever other doctors were recommending (which at the time was nothing), she finally consented.

In the homeopathic interview, I discovered more detail about Dyan's abdominal pain and about various other symptoms she was experiencing. She told me that her abdominal pain extended to her back and that it diminished if she hit it or if she lay on her left side. She told me that she frequently got cramps in her legs before falling asleep and that she often ground her teeth during her sleep. She told me that she loved ice drinks ("the colder, the better"), desired sweets, and was aggravated by eating cabbage. Two characteristics of her personality that, from a homeopathic perspective, would be considered symptoms were that she was offended easily and was stubborn. One other important bit of information helpful to determining her medicine was that she was noticeably overweight.

Although these symptoms may seem unrelated to each other, they actually fit a recognizable pattern to someone knowledgeable about homeopathy. *Calcarea carbonica 200c* (calcium carbonate or chalk) is the medicine I prescribed for her. *Calcarea carbonica* is a very common medicine for people who are overweight, though individualization of the person's totality of symptoms is still necessary for accurate prescribing. The other symptoms listed above also fit *Calcarea carbonica.*

After two weeks, I called Dyan to see if there had been any progress. She said she did not notice anything. When I asked her if she noticed *any* change in her abdominal pain, there was silence. When I repeated the question, she replied that it seemed that the pain had gone away on its own and that she had apparently healed herself. I agreed with her that she had healed herself, but I told her that the medicine might have helped. She still insisted that the medicine had nothing to do with it.

Upon further questioning, I discovered that her leg cramps had gone away, though she was still grinding her teeth and she was still as stubborn as ever.

Two years later, she finally admitted that the homeopathic medicine probably worked after all. Since then, she has been under homeopathic care.

Of particular importance in this case is the fact that homeopathic medicines can be prescribed and can be effective with or without a conventional medical diagnosis. Since homeopathic medicines are prescribed based on the person's symptoms, not from diagnostic categories or presuppositions of organic cause, homeopathy has a real potential for filling a major gap in health care for people whose diagnosis eludes orthodox physicians.

Another lesson from this case is that belief in homeopathy is not necessary for the medicines to be effective. Belief in homeopathy—or whatever treatment one experiences—is no doubt helpful, but it is not a necessary component in the healing process.

A "side effect" of my sister's successful treatment was a change in our physician-father's attitude toward homeopathy. Since it was obvious to him that my sister did not believe in homeopathy, despite its impressive results, he acknowledged that there might be something to it after all. Although some people assume that a homeopath's family is bound to be more receptive to homeopathy than other people, just the opposite can be the case, for obvious reasons of resistance and family dynamics. An informal survey of my fellow homeopaths has convinced me that changing the attitudes of one's own family is generally more difficult than changing the attitudes of strangers. Now that this challenge has been successfully met, I am working on the second most difficult group of people—my neighbors.

Concluding Thoughts

Homeopathy indeed has much to offer to the understanding and treatment of chronic disease. It is sad that most American physicians know virtually nothing about homeopathy and thus cannot even choose whether or not to make use of what it has to offer.

It is particularly sad that most American physicians are so antagonistic to homeopathy that they usually do not believe the patients who tell them that homeopathic medicine cured their chronic
conditions. The cycle of ignorance remains unbroken. Physicians'
common knee-jerk response to such patients is that the cure was
probably a "spontaneous remission" or the medicine was "only
a placebo."

So, if you're tired of experiencing the side effects of conventional drugs and wish to be cured by a "spontaneous remission"
or a "placebo" or whatever, perhaps you should try homeopathy,
too.

Notes

1. Quoted here from Rick Carlson, *The End of Medicine* (New York:
John Wiley, 1975), p. 21.

2. John C. Bailar, III, and Elaine M. Smith, "Progress Against
Cancer?" *New England Journal of Medicine*, 314 (May 8, 1986): 1231.

3. John Cairns, "The Treatment of Diseases and the War Against
Cancer," *Scientific American*, 253 (1985): 59.

4. D. S. Greenberg, "Progress in Cancer Research—Don't Say It
Isn't So," *New England Journal of Medicine*, 292 (1975): 707.

5. Ron Rosenbaum, "Tales from the Cancer Cure Underground,"
New West, November 17, 1980, p. 29.

6. Laura Reif, "Hospitals: How to Get Out Sooner and Stay Out
Longer," *Healthline*, 2 (November 1983): 1–2.

7. G. A. Faich et al., "National Adverse Drug Reaction Surveillance:
1985," *Journal of the American Medical Association*, 257 (April 1987):
2068.

8. National Center for Health Statistics, "National Health Survey,"
Series 10 (1979), pp. 119 and 137, Tables 9 and 14.

9. Ibid.

10. K. Steele et al., "Iatrogenic Illness on a General Medical Service at a University Hospital," *New England Journal of Medicine*, 304
(1981): 638–642.

11. P. A. F. Jansen et al., in *Age and Ageing*, 15 (May 1986): 151.

12. I. Hjermann et al., "Effect of Diet and Smoking Intervention
on the Incidence of Coronary Heart Disease," *Lancet*, 2 (1981): 1303–10.

13. Julian Whitaker, *Reversing Heart Disease* (New York: Warner, 1985).

14. For further information on miasms, see Samuel Hahnemann, *Chronic Diseases* (New Delhi: B. Jain, n.d.); Herbert Roberts, *The Principles and Art of Cure by Homeopathy* (Essex, England: C. W. Daniel, 1942); James Tyler Kent, *Lectures on Homoeopathic Philosophy* (Berkeley: North Atlantic Books, 1979); J. H. Allen, *Chronic Miasms* (New Delhi: B. Jain, n.d.); P. S. Ortega, *Notes on the Miasms* (New Delhi: National Homeopathic Pharmacy, 1980).

15. "Can Aluminum Cause Alzheimer's?" *Wellness Letter* (University of California, Berkeley), 3 (October 1986): 1.

16. Andrew Locke, "A Comparison of Alumina—The Drug Picture—and Alzheimer's Disease—The Disease Picture," *British Homoeopathic Journal*, 73 (April 1984): 92–94.

17. Robin Gibson et al., "Homoeopathic Therapy in Rheumatoid Arthritis: Evaluation by Double-Blind Clinical Trial," *British Journal of Clinical Pharmacology*, 9 (March 1980): 453–459.

18. David Taylor-Reilly, Morag A. Taylor, Charles McSharry, and Tom Aitchison, "Is Homoeopathy a Placebo Response? Controlled Trial of Homoeopathic Potency, with Pollen in Hayfever as Model," *Lancet*, 8514 (October 18, 1986): 881–886.

19. Peter Fisher, "An Experimental Double-Blind Clinical Trial Method in Homoeopathy," *British Homoeopathic Journal*, 75 (July 1986): 142–147.

Additional References

Ornish, Dean. *Stress, Diet, and Your Heart.* New York: Signet, 1984.

Preston, Thomas A. *The Clay Pedestal.* New York: Scribner's, 1981.

Robin, Eugene D. *Medical Care Can Be Dangerous to Your Health.* New York: Harper and Row, 1984.

10

Sports Medicine: Achieving Peak Performance and Healing Injuries Faster with Homeopathic Medicines

Some physicians feel that it is important for people to receive a medical checkup prior to developing an exercise program. Considering the benefits of exercise and the problems that arise from a sedentary lifestyle, it seems more appropriate to seek medical supervision if one chooses *not* to exercise.

There are numerous good reasons to exercise regularly. It can improve heart function and circulation. It can promote the development of stronger bones and muscles. It can help a person to reduce weight. It can lengthen one's endurance and help bodily flexibility. It can promote clearer mental functioning and improve one's emotional health. And some people exercise for the real joy that it gives them. As world marathon champion Ian Thompson said: "I have only to think of putting on my running shoes, and the kinesthetic pleasure of floating starts to come over me."

Whatever the reason one chooses to exercise, there are certain risks involved, too. Injuries are all too common, not just in competitive sports but also in the simple venture of jogging. Joggers, in fact, account for 85 percent of patients' visits to sports doctors. The average runner has 2½ injuries and loses a minimum of seven days of running time per year.[1] According to *Runner's World*, two out of three runners get hurt every year.[2] Considering that there are approximately 25 million Americans who jog, there are a potential 50 million injured legs, knees, or ankles every year.

Not only is there a high injury rate among joggers, but there are lots of injuries in the increasingly popular practice of aerobics. One recent study showed an alarming 75.9 percent injury rate among teachers of aerobics.[3]

In surveying the types of injuries that occur from athletic endeavors, Southern California podiatrist John Pagliano and orthopedic surgeon Douglas Jackson discovered that 45 percent were foot injuries, 25 percent were knee injuries, and 13 percent were lower-leg injuries.[4]

The most common treatment given immediately after an injury is the famous RICE treatment—that is, *R*est, *I*ce, *C*ompression, and *E*levation. This treatment is usually helpful, though athletes often seek additional methods to reduce pain and speed the healing process. Since injuries to professional athletes can hurt or even ruin their careers, and since injuries to average people can prevent them from engaging in their exercise programs, it is certainly understandable that people do whatever they can to get "back on their feet again" as soon as possible.

Some people resort to basic painkillers such as Codeine, Darvon, or Zomax, or stronger ones such as Demerol or Percodan. These drugs are generally effective in reducing the pain one feels, but they do not speed the process of healing. In fact, these drugs simply mask the pain, giving a false sense that there is no injury. And because the person tends to ignore the problem, there is increased risk of further damage to the injured part.

A good example (or, more accurately, a bad example) of using painkillers is in the treatment of shin splints (injuries to muscles that lie alongside the shinbone). Shin splints are one of the most common injuries among people who jog or who do aerobics. They are generally the result of running on hard surfaces. If one does not take care of this injury, or if one continues to utilize the injured part, there is a real possibility that one will develop a stress fracture. Whereas shin splints may last anywhere from one to several weeks when cared for properly, improper care may result in the injury lasting for years. Using painkillers for shin splints may give temporary relief, but may also result in longer-term problems.

Some people use aspirin as a painkiller, but it is ineffective for injuries. It is, however, helpful in reducing muscle soreness after vigorous exercise. Some athletes take aspirin prior to exercising to help prevent this soreness, but aspirin causes increased sweating and urinating, leading to an increased risk of dehydration. Aspirin also tends to decrease the body's ability to clot blood, and thus promotes both internal bleeding of various organs and external bleeding from any cuts, both of which can cause problems for athletes. Various other side effects are also common in frequent users of aspirin. (A homeopathic alternative to aspirin will be discussed later in this chapter.)

Some athletes resort to the use of corticosteroid drugs (for example, cortisone or prednisone) to reduce inflammation from injuries. These drugs are very powerful and are often effective in diminishing pain and in speeding healing when used correctly. However, as with any powerful conventional medications, they can be very dangerous, too, especially when used too frequently. Locally, they can weaken muscle fibers, though this does not lead to a problem unless one receives repeated injections. Effects on the person's overall health may be minimal from a single injection; however, repeated injections can have seriously damaging effects on a person's immune system.

Besides medications, people with injuries may receive various therapeutic measures from sports doctors, chiropractors, physical therapists, massage practitioners, acupuncturists, naturopaths, or other health professionals. These treatments may include massage, heat treatments, traction, therapeutic exercises, ultrasound, electrotherapy, manipulation of joints, orthotics (custom-made arch support), self-hypnosis, acupuncture, acupressure, and, of course, homeopathic medicine.

Homeopathy and Sports Medicine

Football superstar O. J. Simpson, ex-Yankee pitcher Jim Bouton, 1972 National Basketball Association rookie-of-the-year Bob Mac-Adoo, Los Angeles Laker coach Pat Riley, pro golfer Sally Little, and various Olympic athletes spell relief H-O-M-E-O-P-A-T-H-Y. All of them have used homeopathic medicines to relieve injuries or improve their health so that they can perform their best. Since some sports are incredibly competitive, homeopathic medicines offer many people that extra edge that is so important in achieving one's peak performance.

Kate Schmidt, two-time Olympic medalist in javelin throwing, says that "homeopathy can be effective in treating almost anything short of what needs surgery." She notes in particular that she uses homeopathic medicines before and after working out. "I've found," she says, "that homeopathy also helps me to have a good workout by helping my body work more efficiently. It also reduces or even eliminates the typical body aches after a workout."

Homeopathic medicines are not only useful in helping to heal injuries more rapidly, but they can also improve a person's overall health. This strengthening of the body reduces the chances of injury, and, equally important, it improves overall functioning by speeding the healing process when athletes are ill.

Ronald Lawrence, M.D., Ph.D., Assistant Clinical Professor at the UCLA School of Medicine, and consultant to the U.S. Olympic Committee, notes: "Many athletes, like other people, experience respiratory infections, digestive problems, hormonal imbalances, and various other conditions. I have seen homeopathic medicines work exceptionally well in speeding the healing process of these conditions, which allows athletes to work out more efficiently, return to activity more rapidly, and perform at higher levels of competence."

Ex-Yankee pitcher Jim Bouton had an experience with homeopathy that certainly got his attention. "I had a severe case of asthma," he says, "which made it extremely difficult to breathe. I usually need to be hospitalized. A friend gave me the name of a homeopath who gave me a medicine which worked incredibly rapidly. Within twenty-four hours, my breathing was completely cleared, and I was on the mound that next day . . . as the winning pitcher."

Treating injuries with homeopathic medicine is relatively easy. Although chronic disease requires strict individualization of a homeopathic medicine, the medicines that are commonly effective in treating people's injuries are fairly consistent, because what one person needs to heal an injury is generally what others also need. In contrast, the origin of chronic diseases varies so much from person to person that more individualized care is a necessity.

Before discussing the specifics of homeopathic sports medicine, I should point out that homeopaths will not use only homeopathic medicines in the treatment of their patients. They may utilize non-drug treatments similar to those given by professionals who specialize in sports medicine, or they may refer their patients to non-homeopathic specialists. But they generally will not prescribe as many conventional medications and, whenever possible, will rely on homeopathic remedies to relieve their patients' pain and stimulate their healing processes.

Nonprofessionals can also learn to treat themselves for many common injuries. Although chronic conditions should receive the attention of a trained homeopath, laypersons are often surprised by their ability to help themselves with homeopathic medicines.

Arnica (mountain daisy) is the most common homeopathic medicine in sports medicine. It is used for the initial shock and trauma of various injuries, and it is of great benefit in the treatment of sore muscles from overexertion or the achiness that comes from exercising muscles that are not often utilized. *Arnica* can be used before and after a workout to prevent the muscle aches. It has been dubbed the "homeopath's aspirin" for its effectiveness in preventing and treating sore muscles after workouts.

Whit Reeves, a New Mexico acupuncturist who utilizes homeopathic medicine and who specializes in sports medicine, has found that homeopathy is invaluable in marathons. "Not only does *Arnica* reduce muscle aches," he says, "it also diminishes the chances of cramping, swelling, and tissue injury. Since it is impractical to give an acupuncture treatment during a marathon, I can give my patients who run marathons a quick dose of *Arnica* at one of the water stations."

Arnica can be taken internally or applied externally in an ointment, lotion, or mineral oil base. The British cycling team that competed in the 1984 Olympics in Los Angeles used homeopathic medicines as one of their secret weapons. Jim Hendry, Director of Racing for the British Cycling Federation, noted: "I first learnt about *Arnica Ointment* from a coach who used it for gymnasts who were always banging their legs on the parallel bars. I was pleased with the initial results and decided to introduce it with all the National Teams."[5]

Bart Flick, an orthopedic surgeon in private practice in Ville Platte, Louisiana, notes: "The sooner I can get a dose of *Arnica* to a person with a ligament or soft tissue contusion, the faster there is resolution of the problem. *Arnica* cuts the healing time in half or less." Dr. Flick also added: "I've seen people use *Arnica lotion*, and it diminishes pain very rapidly. A problem is created, however, when the person forgets about the pain and goes about his or her daily business. These people may wash themselves, including the injured part, unconsciously washing off the *Arnica lotion*. The pain then returns until they reapply more. I am very confident that every orthopedic physician and, in fact, every physician will use *Arnica* in the near future."

If there is a collection of blood (a hematoma) along with a muscle injury or with any type of sprain or strain, homeopaths give *Bellis perennis* (daisy). When the person sprains his or her ankle, and swelling with blood occurs under the skin, *Ledum* (marsh tea) is the remedy of choice. If there is still any soreness after this blood has been absorbed by the body, *Arnica* is given.

Some athletes experience burning pains in their muscles after heavy workouts. This is particularly common for weightlifters. These pains are often successfully treated with *Apis* (crushed bee) or *Arnica*.

Rhus tox (poison ivy) is one of the key medicines for sprains, especially the type of sprain in which one experiences pain upon initial motion but less pain in continuing to move. Sprained ankles or wrists, Achilles tendonitis, and plantarfasciitis (inflammation of the band of tissue under the foot's arch) are especially amenable to effective treatment with *Rhus tox. Anacardium* (marking nut) is another medicine for Achilles tendonitis, especially when the person does not have the aggravation of pain when moving that is so typical of those who need *Rhus tox. Bryonia* (wild hops) is commonly given to people with sprains when pain is experienced on any type of motion of the injured part. Sprains that seem to heal very slowly should be treated with *Zinc*.

One of the major homeopathic medicines effective in treating sprained hamstring muscles (those muscles in the back of the upper leg) is *Ammonium muriaticum* (ammonium chloride).

Ruta (rue) is a superb medicine for injuries to the periosteum (bone covering), especially in the knee and elbow. It is an effective medicine for tennis elbow and golfer's elbow, though it has been said that another effective "medicine" for these conditions is a tennis or golf lesson.

Ruta is also given for shin splints. *Rhus tox* is another commonly prescribed remedy for shin splints, especially when the person says that the pain is worse after rather than during a run. Janet Zand, a homeopath and acupuncturist in Los Angeles who treats many athletes, has found that *Nux vomica* (poison nut) and *Carbo veg* (vegetable charcoal), when given in alternating doses, are often helpful for shin splints, too. These medicines are more commonly known to homeopaths for their ability to treat digestive symptoms and are not normally used in the treatment of shin splints. Dr. Zand, however, has noted that the stomach meridian runs adjacent to the shin bone (the tibia), which may explain how medicines that strengthen the digestive process may also help other parts of the body.

Chondromalacia, commonly called "runner's knee," is a frequent condition among persons who jog or do aerobics. It is an irritation of the undersurface of the kneecap. Homeopaths can treat this condition effectively with any of a variety of medicines that must be individualized. The most common are *Arnica, Rhus tox, Rhododendron,* and *Ruta.*

Arnica is considered at the early stage, when runner's knee has not yet become a chronic problem, when the pain is primarily the result of overuse of the legs, and when it is not severe. *Rhus tox* is considered when the recurrent pain is worse on initial motion, whereas *Rhododendron* is indicated when the pain decreases on initial motion. *Ruta* is of value in true chondromalacia, in which the person develops unstable knees when they walk as well as run. The pain of persons needing *Ruta* will be noticeably aggravated when they go down stairs. Besides *Ruta,* orthotic foot control, rest, and special exercises are necessary for optimal treatment.

Another medicine that is occasionally used for runner's knee is *Apis.* This remedy is especially helpful when there is an obvious sensation of heat with the knee inflammation, and when the person's pain is aggravated by warm applications and reduced by cold applications. Dr. Zand has found that alternating the use of *Apis* and *Ruta* is a particularly effective treatment for runner's knee. She recommends taking each of these medicines four times a day for three days; *Apis* should be taken first, and *Ruta* should be taken an hour later. Finally, Dr. Zand notes that if none of these medicines works, *Calcarea phosphorica* (calcium phosphate) may be helpful.

Although homeopathic medicines are generally very effective in treating runner's knee, some people will need surgery. Those people with recurrent runner's knee should seek the attention of a sports medicine specialist and/or orthopedic surgeon.

Mag phos (phosphate of magnesia) is indicated for tight muscles and cramping that are alleviated by heat, while *Colocynthis* (bitter cucumber) is given for a similar condition relieved by pressure. These two medicines are also helpful for sciatica pains, though there are several other potential homeopathic medicines that may be preferable. (Care from a trained homeopath is always recommended for persons with sciatica.) *Cuprum metallicum* (copper) is another common medicine for cramps, especially in the calves or soles.

Hypericum (St. John's wort) is a medicine par excellence for injuries with shooting pains. Such conditions indicate trauma to a nerve, and *Hypericum* works rapidly both to diminish such pains and to heal the injury. It is often also indicated for injuries to the toes, since many nerves end there. It is also indicated for back injuries in which there are shooting pains. But *Hypericum* is not helpful for back pain, except that from injury.

Homeopathic medicines may contribute to the healing of back injuries, though massage, physical therapy, and chiropractic or osteopathic manipulation can also be helpful. *Rhus tox* is indicated when pain is aggravated by initial motion or cold, wet weather but relieved by continued motion. *Arnica* is valuable for a bruised sensation in the back that arises from straining muscles by exercise or lifting an object. Other homeopathic medicines should also be considered.

Symphytum (comfrey) is extremely valuable for the common fracture, while *Silica* (silica) is indicated when there are small bone chips from a fracture. *Bryonia* is given for fractured ribs, since this medicine has an affinity for the chest in general.

Besides the various serious injuries that homeopathic medicines can treat effectively, homeopathy can also help what is perhaps the most common complaint of people just beginning their exercise program: blisters! *Calendula* (marigold) in an ointment, lotion, or mineral oil base is highly effective in healing blisters. One can apply *Calendula* directly to the blister or first puncture it with a sterilized needle, drain it without tearing or removing the skin, and then apply *Calendula* to the surface.

Calendula is also effective in the treatment of various cuts, scrapes, and even burns. The organic iodine in this herb helps to prevent infection, and its other nutrients nurture the injured part back to health.

Despite the many ways in which individuals can learn to treat themselves effectively with homeopathic medicine, there are times when professional homeopathic care is necessary. Such care is recommended when a person has recurrent symptoms of an injury or when a person gets injured easily (for example, is susceptible to frequently sprained ankles, or develops muscle achiness from the slightest exertion; these conditions suggest an internal problem, not simply an injury). Some homeopathic medicines may temporarily relieve a person's pain when a deeper-acting medicine may be necessary to promote a true healing.

Dr. Hans Kraus, a specialist in sports medicine, has asserted that fifteen minutes of exercise causes the heart to beat 100–120 times a minute, which has a measurably greater relaxing effect on the body than 400 milligrams of the best tranquilizers available.[6] Since many of us who exercise seek the many benefits that it offers, it is good to know that there are homeopathic medicines that can help us to heal from its injuries and side effects.

Sherrie Moore, holder of the women's transcontinental world record in cycling, is another athlete who is impressed with the results of the homeopathic medicines she has taken. "The medicines offer an immediate cure of so many common injuries," she says. "I don't understand homeopathy or how the medicines work, but I do know that they work and that they don't cause any harm."

Podiatrist and sports medicine specialist Steven Subotnick has authored two books on his field in association with *Runner's World*. Ironically, at the time he was writing these, he was unfamiliar with homeopathy, and consequently he was commonly recommending conventional medications, since he thought nothing else was available. Dr. Subotnick now notes: "I give homeopathic medicines to virtually every patient I see. They work incredibly well, and I just wish I knew about them a long time ago."

Whether one plays competitive sports or not, homeopathy helps people to become winners—and it makes the process of winning a lot less painful.

Notes

1. Matthew King, "The Chronic Boom," *City Sports*, October 1986, p. 45.
2. Steven I. Subotnick, *Cures for Common Running Injuries* (New York: Collier, 1979), p. xi.
3. King, "Chronic Boom," p. 48.
4. Ibid.
5. "Arnica at the Olympics," *Homeopathy Today*, Summer 1984, p. 25.
6. Hans Kraus, *Sports Injuries* (Chicago: Playboy, 1981), p. 5.

Additional References

Bachman, David C., and Marilynn Preston. *Dear Dr. Jock . . . The People's Guide to Sports and Fitness*. New York: Dutton, 1980.

Benjamin, Ben E., and Gale Borden. *Listen to Your Pain*. New York: Penguin, 1984.

Priestman, Kathleen Gordon. "Homoeopathic Injury Remedies." *British Homoeopathic Journal*, 48 (July 1959): 281–289.

Reuben, Carolyn. "Jock's Traps: Help for Sports Injuries." *L.A. Weekly*, May 31, 1985, p. 75.

Schwartz, William H. *Homoeopathic Medical Treatment of Wounds and Injuries*. New Delhi: Harjeet, n.d.

Shangold, Mona, and Gabe Mirkin. *The Complete Sports Medicine Book for Women.* New York: Simon and Schuster, 1985.

Wolpa, Mark E. *The Sports Medicine Guide.* New York: Leisure Press, 1983.

11

Psychological Problems: Treating Mind and Body

Charles Frederick Menninger, M.D., the founder of the famous mental health facility named after him, the Menninger Clinic, was actually a homeopathic physician. He joined the American Institute of Homeopathy in 1894 and shortly thereafter became the head of his local medical society. Dr. Menninger was such an advocate of homeopathy that he once said: "Homeopathy is wholly capable of satisfying the therapeutic demands of this age better than any other system or school of medicine."[1]

Hahnemann's name is not referred to in texts on the history of psychology, nor is his name recognized in psychology today. And yet, even before Hahnemann developed the homeopathic science, he made important contributions to mental health care. In the late 1700s, insanity was considered possession by demons. The insane were regarded as wild animals, and treatment was essentially punishment. Hahnemann was one of the few physicians who perceived mental illness as a disease that required humane treatment. He opposed the practice of chaining mental patients, granted respect and human dignity to them, and recommended simple rest and relaxation. Although this type of care may seem obvious today, it was revolutionary in its time.

Present-day historians and psychiatrists recognize that the treatment of the insane was often barbaric in the past. But these experts are not just recalling the past of the 1700s or 1800s; mental health care of just the past several decades was filled with abuses. The mentally ill were injected with malaria in the hope that the fever would burn out their insanity. Insulin was given to schizophrenics, even though it seemed to diminish their symptoms only when given in very high, sometimes lethal, doses. In the 1950s, between forty and fifty thousand prefrontal lobotomies were performed (in this operation, the frontal lobe of the brain is incised, usually leaving the patient in a zombielike state).[2] Neuroleptic drugs such as Thorazine (chlorprozine), Haldol (haloperidol), and Prolexine (flufenazine) were and still are frequently, sometimes too frequently, given to psychotic patients. These drugs may cause severe acute muscular spasms and bizarre posturing, and may eventually lead to Parkinsonian syndrome.

These various treatments are now either outdated or have been moderated, and yet it remains questionable if modern psychiatric care is optimum.

Modern Psychiatric Care

Although treatment for the mentally ill has progressed in the past few decades, it is still hard not to think that some of the psychiatric care offered today will be considered barbaric in the distant or even near future.

Mental illness is certainly one of the major health problems today. The National Institute of Mental Health estimated in 1984 that one in every five Americans has a mental disorder.[3] This same study revealed that, during a six-month period, 8.3 percent of Americans suffered from an anxiety disorder (including phobias), 6.4 percent had a substance abuse (alcohol or drug) problem, and 6 percent had an affective (mood) disorder.

For a long time, psychiatrists and psychologists had great difficulty in defining what constituted mental illness and what differentiated one type of illness from another. In 1980, the American Psychiatric Association published the *Diagnostic and Statistical Manual of Mental Disorders* (Third Edition), usually referred to as the *DSM-III*. This text has become the official guide to defining mental disease categories. Although the *DSM-III* presents the most exacting information presently available on mental illness,

Dr. Jerrold Maxmen, a Columbia University psychiatrist, has noted that "*DSM-III* shows how little psychiatrists actually know about mental disorders. . . . Because solid data doesn't exist for so many of these topics [diseases], *DSM-III* spotlights the enormous gaps in factual information about mental disorders."[4]

Despite the advances in the ability of psychiatrists and psychologists to diagnose mental illness, it is not always clear that such diagnoses give us greater understanding of psychological disorders, nor do the diagnoses necessarily teach us how to cure the disorders. The German philosopher Immanuel Kant reminded us of the limitations of diagnosis when he said: "Physicians think they are doing something for you by labeling what you have as a disease."

During the past century, mental health professionals have debated the nature of mental illness. They have asked: to what degree is mental illness biological or organic and to what degree is it psychosocial? Until recently, most psychiatrists took one side or the other on this issue. Today, however, there is a consensus among psychiatrists that, generally speaking, biological factors primarily determine the *type* of symptoms of disorder that a person experiences (for example, delusions or insomnia), while psychosocial factors are primarily responsible for the *content* and *meaning* of these symptoms.

Psychiatrists tend to use medications to deal with the biological aspects of psychological problems and to use psychological therapies to treat the psychosocial condition. Their determination of what drug to use is based on their understanding of brain function. Nerve cells transmit messages by sending electrical impulses and chemicals called neurotransmitters to one another. This action triggers other nerve cells to fire messages or to inhibit this firing, depending on the frequency and intensity of the message transmitted and the sensitivity of the nerve cells' receptors.

Psychiatric medications are chosen to influence these mechanisms. People with schizophrenia, for example, are found to have nerve cell receptors that are hypersensitive to certain neurotransmitters, and thus these cells fire too easily. *Chlorpromazine* (Thorazine), *trifluoperazine* (Stelazine), and *haloperidol* (Haldol) are some of the antipsychotic medications given to schizophrenics to help reduce this hypersensitivity and to calm them.

Psychiatrists believe that severe depression results from a decrease in receptivity to certain neurotransmitters; thus, medications are prescribed to increase this receptivity. Tricyclic antidepressant medications, most commonly *amitriptyline* (Elavil) and *imipramine* (Tofranil), are thought to have this stimulating action. Monoamine oxidase (MAO) inhibitors are also given for depression, in part because they prevent the breakdown of some neurotransmitters, and in part because they seem to relieve symptoms of depressive patients. Amphetamines are sometimes still given to depressive patients, especially the elderly; however, it has been discovered that cells tend to develop a tolerance for and an addiction to such drugs, requiring increasingly stronger doses of them to have an effect.

Despite the simplicity of these explanations for why psychiatric medications are prescribed, nature is not always as unidimensional as our explanations of it. Neurotransmitters not only affect nerve function but also directly influence hormones. By intervening in the delicate balance of brain chemistry, drugs can cause significant physiological disruptions. For example, one might assume that the body is physiologically underactive during severe depression. In actual fact, the adrenal glands become hyperactive, producing excessive amounts of cortisol, the body's principal "stress" hormone. Various neurological, cardiovascular, digestive, hematologic (blood), and allergic symptoms are side effects of most antidepressive drugs.

The MAO inhibitors cause such a disruption of the body that many common foods and drinks (aged cheese, yogurt, beer, chocolate, raisins, coffee, yeast products, and others) have to be avoided, since their ingestion can cause high blood pressure and, in a small number of cases, death.[6]

There are 10 trillion nerve cells in the brain that govern sensing, thinking, and feeling.[7] Despite the varying functions of different groups of nerve cells, their interdependent and synergistic nature creates a highly complex working whole that is literally impossible to comprehend fully. Predictably, psychiatrists have

had limited success trying to alter certain improperly functioning parts without directly disturbing brain chemistry and physiological processes.

Author Lyall Watson has noted: "If the brain were so simple
that we could understand it, we would be so simple that we couldn't
understand it." And acknowledging the complexity of the brain
and of human behavior, Albert Einstein once said: "How difficult
it is! How much more difficult psychology is than physics."

Despite the fact that psychiatric drugs often have serious side
effects, especially when given over long periods of time, and despite
the additional fact that they do not actually cure mental illness,
these drugs still serve an important function. Since approximately
15 percent of people with severe depression commit suicide,[8] methods to alleviate depression and thereby reduce the chances of
suicide are certainly needed. If, however, there are alternatives
to these methods, it is certainly prudent to consider them. Dr.
Charles Frederick Menninger reminds us that "it is imperative that
we *exhaust* the homeopathic healing art before resorting to any
other mode of treatment, if we wish to accomplish the greatest
success possible."[9]

The Homeopathic
Understanding of Mental Illness

The homeopathic understanding of health is intimately connected
to its understanding of the mind in general. Homeopaths do not
separate the mind and body in the usual way; they generally
assume that body and mind are dynamically interconnected and
directly influence each other. This acknowledgment of the inter-
connectedness of body and mind is not simply a vague, impractical concept. Homeopaths base virtually every homeopathic prescription on the physical and psychological symptoms of the sick
person. Psychological symptoms often play a primary role in the
selection of the correct medicine.

Trying to determine whether a person's mental state caused
his physical disease or vice versa is rarely helpful in discovering
the correct homeopathic medicine. Most of the time, this determination is moot. Instead, the homeopath seeks to find a medicine

that matches the totality of the person's physical and psychological symptoms, irrespective of "which came first."

The "which came first" issue is much more complex and deceptive than one might initially suppose. Most of us have probably said at one time or another that we got a headache or some other symptoms after getting angry, being depressed, or becoming fearful, and that this emotion "caused" the headache. The emotional stress, however, may be only the veritable "straw on the camel's back" that results in the collapse of the camel (or in the development of the headache). This collapse was not necessarily "caused" by the straw, but may have resulted because the camel was already carrying a load of 500 pounds—that is, because we were concomitantly experiencing various physical, environmental, and other stresses in our life.

Too often we assume that something that happens close to the time we develop symptoms is "the cause" of our problem. It is always easier, however, to look for the effects of causes than for the causes of effects. In actuality, what we assume to be the "cause" is probably only another effect or another stress. The "cause" of a phenomenon is not so simple and may not ever be known. The Greek philosopher Democritus understood this paradox when he said that he would rather understand one cause than be King of Persia.

Contemporary psychologist Lawrence LeShan has also questioned the value of finding the "original cause" of a mental disorder. "One does not put out a forest fire," he notes, "by extinguishing the match that started it."

The homeopathic alternative to treating psychological and physical diseases is to assume that mind and body are undeniably connected and that a microdose must be individually prescribed, based on the totality of the sick person's symptoms.

From a homeopathic point of view, the prevalence of mental illness in our society is not simply the result of living in a fast-paced, stressful society, but also derives from our medical care system having effectively suppressed various physical illnesses. Homeopaths assert that by treating symptoms as "causes" rather than as "effects," conventional medicine masks the symptoms without curing the underlying disease process. Homeopaths theorize that, worse still, the suppression of symptoms forces the disease process deeper into the organism, so that it then manifests itself in more severe physical pathology and more serious psychological disorders.

Homeopaths and biologists alike acknowledge that living organisms respond to stresses in ways that primarily allow for survival. Organisms will protect their most vital processes first. Homeopaths therefore assume that a person's mental state is vital for survival insofar as it governs the state of awareness that makes decisions on how to respond to stressful or life-threatening situations. The organism will protect the deepest psychological level most strongly and will first externalize various superficial emotions. Likewise on a physical level, certain vital organs, especially the brain and the heart, will be protected before other organs.

Homeopaths operate on the assumption that the organism creates the best possible response, based on its present abilities, to whatever stresses it is experiencing. Because homeopaths view symptoms as adaptive efforts of the organism to respond to stress or infection, they assume that efforts to control or suppress these defensive reactions can only lead to more serious symptoms. The evidence supporting this assumption can be found in any pharmacology text that lists the side effects of drugs. It becomes immediately apparent that the side effects of drugs are often more serious than the condition they are treating. And predictably, these side effects include various acute and chronic mental symptoms. A classic example of this phenomenon can be observed in the use of corticosteroids (cortisone and prednisone) to suppress skin eruptions and asthmatic attacks. In addition to the various side effects of these drugs, corticosteroids are also known to induce depression and even psychosis, which diminish when the drug dosage is reduced or stopped. (More detail about the curative process and the suppression of disease can be found in the "Understanding the Healing Process" section of Chapter 1 and in the "Homeopaths' Understanding of Chronic Disease" section of Chapter 9.)

Psychological symptoms, too, are regarded by homeopaths as ways in which a person is trying to adapt to biological and psychosocial stresses. Such symptoms should not be suppressed unless this is medically necessary. Instead, a homeopathic medicine should be individually prescribed, based on the totality of the person's symptoms. The correct homeopathic medicine will catalyze a healing process that will raise the person's overall level of health. To complement the prescription, good homeopaths will provide some psychotherapeutic support based on homeopathic principles to be discussed shortly. Of course, when appropriate, homeopaths will also refer clients to various other health practitioners.

The Homeopathic Treatment of Psychological Problems

Several schools of psychology categorize people by certain psychological or characterological types. Other health professionals working in medicine, genetics, or sports categorize people by various "body types." Homeopaths, in contrast, acknowledge certain "bodymind" types. They determine their medicines based on the *constellation* of physical and psychological symptoms.

Choosing the correct homeopathic medicine is at once a highly systematic and an artful process. Edward C. Whitmont, M.D., one of the founders of the New York Jungian Training Center and a homeopath since the 1940s, has written eloquently about the homeopathic bodymind types. In his book *Psyche and Substance: Essays on Homeopathy in the Light of Jungian Psychology*, Dr. Whitmont describes a dozen key medicines that homeopaths use, the role that each of these substances plays in nature, the chemistry of each substance and how it acts the way it does, the symptoms that it is known to cause in human beings when given in a toxic dose, and the bodymind type it is known to treat and cure.[10]

In a similar fashion, Catherine Coulter, a homeopath in Washington, D.C., has written *Portraits of Homoeopathic Medicines*, in which she describes the bodymind types in the light of well-known characters in history, in literature, and even in comic books and comic strips.[11]

In order to give a sense of some specifics of these homeopathic typologies, I will describe two medicines, *Arsenicum album* (arsenic) and *Nux vomica* (poison nut). The following descriptions are brief summaries. For more detailed information, consult the books by Whitmont and Coulter, articles by Vithoulkas,[12] and various materia medicas.[13]

The person who needs *Arsenicum* is an overanxious, restless, fearful, perfectionist type of person. He or she has a driven nature and suffers from a fussy meticulousness, which creates a high-strung and nervous individual. In general, people needing *Arsenicum* tend to assume that there are hostile forces at work in the world and that they must work vigilantly against them. They have a deep-seated insecurity, from which develops a dependency on others, a possessiveness of objects and people, a tendency toward fastidiousness, and deeply felt anxieties and fears. They may have various anxieties and fears, especially about their health, their future, and their financial status, all of which are heightened when they are alone and diminished when they are with others. To reduce the chances of things going wrong, they become overconscientious. They overprepare for everything and are inordinately fastidious.

Physically, the person who needs *Arsenicum* is usually thin, fine-haired, delicate skinned, with a pale or alabaster complexion. They perspire easily and profusely and are extremely sensitive to factors in the external environment. They are particularly sensitive to any exposure to cold and feel better from most forms of heat. They tend to experience burning pains that are relieved by warm applications; and if they have those pains in the stomach, these are relieved by warm drinks. Milk, fruit, ice cream, and alcohol may aggravate digestive or other symptoms. Most commonly, their physical and psychological symptoms will be particularly apparent at midnight and shortly after.

The symptoms that typify the *Arsenicum* type are often seen in insomniacs. Because the symptoms of *Arsenicum* are worse late at night, and because these people tend to be perfectionistic, they usually require things to be "just right" in order to fall asleep. Part of their hypersensitivity to the environment lies in a sensitivity to noise—any noise.

Part of their overconscientious nature is an anxiety about health. People who need *Arsenicum*, are often hypochondriacs. They have many, many symptoms; and even though they may have had these for a long time, they still want the practitioner to get rid of them immediately. As a result of this anxiety, they tend to go to a variety of doctors and usually try many types of alternative therapies. These people also tend to become addicted to various pain relievers or other medications that temporarily diminish their pain. Also, because of their anxious and restless nature, they may use drugs or alcohol to slow them down and help them relax.

Arsenicum is also a common medicine given to people with anorexic tendencies. People who need *Arsenicum* tend to have anxieties about the food they eat, sometimes thinking that all food is toxic and that they should not eat at all. Another part of their personality that fosters anorexia is their perfectionistic nature, which tends to encourage a thinner and thinner waistline.

Nux vomica has several similarities to *Arsenicum*, but more distinct differences. People who need *Nux* are hurried and impulsive, like those who need *Arsenicum*, but *Nux* people are more prone to irritability, anger, and maliciousness. Even those *Nux* people who have learned to control their rage tend to feel a hyper-irritability and anger inside themselves struggling to be expressed. They are dissatisfied, rarely content, hypercritical of others, impatient, and jealous. They are very competitive. They will compete compulsively even in certain games or job situations in which competition is not appropriate.

Like people who need *Arsenicum*, *Nux* people will be fastidious. But whereas *Arsenicum* people will usually become anxious and nervous as they try to hold in their disgust for messes, *Nux* people will often get irritated and visibly angered by lack of order and cleanliness.*

People who need *Nux* tend to be extremely self-reliant, a distinct difference from those who need *Arsenicum*. *Nux* people will overemphasize achievement, to such a degree that their lives will become dominated by their work. They will take on greater responsibility than they are capable of, becoming increasingly ir-

---

*It should be noted that homeopaths recognize that a person can be neat, orderly, and fastidious in a healthy way. However, whenever homeopaths refer to fastidiousness as a symptom, they are referring to a state in which the individual is overly concerned about cleanliness and order.

ritable and demanding.

Classically, people who need *Nux* represent what is called in psychology the "authoritarian personality."[14] They want to force things their own way. To achieve security they adopt a powerful authority and demand that those in inferior positions submit to it. Whitmont describes them as perfect bureaucrats. They are also rigidly moralistic and will condemn others who violate *Nux*'s moral code. They repress their own socially disapproved tendencies and project them onto others.

Nux people also have a soft side. They are sentimental and may cry from listening to certain music or seeing beautiful objects. And despite a rough exterior, they cannot stand the least pain. They may cry even after a bout of anger. Since they cannot tolerate the least opposition, they may cry from frustration. Despite this occasional tendency to weep, some people who need *Nux* often find it impossible to cry.

Physically, people who require *Nux* may be husky, solid, and muscular, or they may be lean, bent forward, and withered. They are physically and emotionally irritated by exposure to cold, drafts, noise, and light. Their worst time of day is upon waking, and it usually takes them an hour or so to wake. They sometimes feel an urge to take a nap. If they are accidentally awakened from this nap, they become highly irritated. They may suffer from insomnia because of their very active minds, which constantly ruminate about the many irons they have in the fire.

They tend to overeat, with cravings for fats, spicy foods, and milk. They may experience various digestive and nervous symptoms that are aggravated by foods that they tend to crave, especially milk, meat, fats, and coffee. Commonly, they will be constipated and have much gas.

Typically, people who need *Nux* sustain their hyperactive nature by drinking coffee, imbibing alcohol, and taking various stimulants. They are therefore prone to alcoholism, drug abuse, and malnutrition. They may be friendly when they are sober; however, when they are drunk or high, they tend to be abusive, cruel, and violent. They will ridicule and scorn others. They thus have tendencies toward spouse and child abuse. They also have strong sexual desires, and they tend to demand much from their sexual partner. Their strong sexual desires, if they are men, may lead them to rape. However, if they have drunk too much or taken too many drugs, they may become impotent, and this may persist even after the effects of the substance have worn off.

People who need *Nux* also have classic "Type A" behavior. They are prone to being workaholics and will often demand a similar level of commitment to work from others. As a result of this hyperactivity, they tend to become hypertensive and are therefore prone to heart disease.

Arsenicum and *Nux* are two of the many homeopathic medicines used to treat people suffering from psychological and physical problems. Homeopaths commonly treat people with acute and chronic psychological disorders, including depression, anxieties and phobias, and emotional and mental states of confusion. Homeopaths also commonly treat people with substance abuse problems.

The late Dr. Jack Cooper was the Chief Psychiatrist for seventeen years at New York's Westchester County Prison and Jail. Although he did not initially use homeopathic medicines at his work in the prison, he was very impressed with the results he received when he finally began to do so. He found that the prisoners he was treating with homeopathic medicines were becoming better able to cope with the withdrawal of drugs and alcohol. He also noted that for several years there were no suicides in the prison, whereas both before he began using the medicines and after he left, there were several suicides every year. Dr. Cooper found that the homeopathic medicines were having dramatic effects on the prisoners' physical and mental health. And of personal significance to Dr. Cooper, he found that his work was no longer frustrating, but rewarding and worthwhile.

Dr. Cooper's practice outside the prison included the treatment of many alcoholics. He conducted an informal study of alcoholics treated with homeopathic medicines. As a way to measure the effects of these medicines and to diminish the possible effects that his own presence may have created, he did not actually see the patients himself in most cases. Instead, he talked to a loved one or relative who intimately knew the alcoholic's physical and psychological symptoms. Of the approximately thirty patients in the study, Dr. Cooper found a 50 percent cure rate, which he defined as a significantly decreased desire for alcohol and the ability to drink socially without excessive physical or psychological symptoms.[15]

Homeopathy actually has a long history of successful treatment of various psychological disorders. In 1874, the first public institution for the homeopathic treatment of the insane was opened in New York state: the Middletown Asylum for the Insane (later called the State Homeopathic Hospital, at Middletown). Comparing the rate of discharge from conventional versus homeopathic mental hospitals in New York state between 1883 and 1890, we find that an average of 30 percent of patients were discharged from conventional hospitals every year, whereas 50 percent of patients in homeopathic hospitals were discharged. Although one can quibble about these statistics for one reason or another, it is much harder to rationalize away the fact that the death rate in conventional mental hospitals was 33 percent higher than that at homeopathic mental hospitals.[16]

By 1899, seven states in the United States had public mental hospitals under homeopathic supervision, and two of these states had more than one.[17]

More recently, two British homeopaths evaluated 120 cases of various neurotic disorders in 1953. Their overall improvement rate was 79 percent after six months, an impressive statistic when one considers that most of their patients had been ill for at least a year, and many for several years.[18]

Psychotherapy: Homeopathic Style

Too often, people assume that psychological problems require psychological solutions. Since some psychological symptoms arise from physiological processes (and vice versa), it is of value to treat the sick person holistically. A holistic approach is inherent in homeopathic care.

A homeopath prescribes the individually chosen medicine for the sick person, but he or she may do more than this. When appropriate, a homeopath will provide basic information on nutrition, exercise, stress management, and social and environmental determinants of health and disease. A homeopath may also counsel the person to help him deal with the emotional and mental state he is experiencing.

Today, many modern psychoanalysts utilize homeopathic-like perspectives and practices. In contrast to some philosophical theories that assume that human nature is essentially destructive and perverted, integral to homeopathy and many psychoanalytic practices is the assumption that human nature is basically creative and that the organism has implicit self-healing capabilities. Symptoms, including psychological ones, are presumed to be ways that the bodymind is trying to adapt to and to deal creatively with various internal and external stresses.

Some very simple psychotherapeutic processes that might be considered "homeopathic" in their approach are "paradoxical intention"[19] and therapeutic double-bind,[20] which try to dislodge the symptom and thus to set a curative process in motion. In these cases, the therapist actually *encourages* the patient to pretend to experience the problematic emotional state. For instance, if a person has a phobia of snakes, he or she is asked to pretend to see a snake and to pretend to feel afraid. This method is considered effective if the person is sometimes unable to produce the fear at will and then is less susceptible to having the phobia at other times.

In another form of paradoxical intention the therapist encourages the patient to exaggerate the emotional or behavioral problem. Milton Erickson gave a classic example of this strategy when he described a boy who sucked his thumb. Rather than discouraging the child from this behavior, Erickson expressed unmistakable concern that the child was not giving equal attention to his other fingers. Erickson asked the child to begin sucking them. Shortly after this suggestion, the child stopped sucking his thumb altogether.[21]

Psychotherapies that recognize the importance of accepting rather than denying one's emotions are an obvious first step toward a "homeopathic" cure. Engaging with and expressing those emotions is the second step. The energy blocked by habituated responses and long-term traumas is thus freed cathartically. The symptoms are transformed in an overall revitalization of the individual's healing capacities.

This approach is certainly more in line with homeopathic

thinking than shortcut methods that define an ideal way of being and encourage patients to act in a specific, prescribed way. Simple rational analysis of emotional processes is likewise an inadequate way of dealing with structures and energies that are unconscious and go to the root of the organism. Behavior modification strategies that primarily change the way one acts but do not affect the underlying tendencies that led to that behavior in the first place are another clearly "unhomeopathic" therapy. And therapeutic measures that palliate extreme symptoms may only temporarily compensate for problems, not cure them.*

Some principles of gestalt therapy are also quite homeopathic. As the name itself implies (*gestalt* means a unified whole), gestalt therapy is a way of looking at a specific problem *in the context* of the whole person. Rather than treating a problem as extraneous to the person and simply trying to change it, gestalt therapists (and therapists from various similar schools of thought as well) encourage their patients to become more aware of themselves in toto and to transform their whole being. If, for example, a person has a sexual problem, the gestalt therapist, like the homeopath, will not understand the problem as only a "sexual problem" but as "a problem of the whole person."

Modern psychoanalysts, like homeopaths, understand that symptoms are not "the problem" but only manifestations of the problem. Sigmund Freud laid the groundwork for this perspective by uncovering the sublimated and unconscious nature of psychological disorders and the manner in which they are expressed. Carl Jung extended this perspective by showing how those sublimated psychological patterns also contain symbolic representations of transpersonal unconscious materials. Wilhelm Reich showed how these patterns are locked into actual physical states. In general, the psychoanalytical process involves the patient in reexperiencing those unconscious dynamic elements that lie at the basis of the pathology. This recreating or mimicking of an original submerged experience is clearly homeopathic-like in the largest sense.

The awareness of the dynamic complexity of symptoms is

---

*Just because a psychotherapeutic intervention is "unhomeopathic" does not mean it does not have an equal value or efficacy in specific cases.

shared by homeopathy and psychoanalysis. Although most classic homeopathic texts contain an outdated psychological terminology, the very basis of homeopathic medicine comprises a sophisticated psychoanalytic framework. More recent homeopathic texts correct this problem,* and the best homeopaths are often excellent psychotherapists.

Still, homeopaths have much to learn from the field of psychology. Too often homeopaths try to obtain information about a person's psyche by asking such direct questions as "What fears do you have? What makes you angry? What types of things make you cry?" Homeopaths obviously have to learn more sophisticated means not only of getting but of interpreting this information and distinguishing real character from affect-oriented and ego-oriented character.

Of course, the field of psychology has much to learn from homeopathy, too. Hering's Law of Cure is an invaluable assessment tool for the progress of treatment. The emphasis in homeopathy on the minimum dose will encourage therapists to find the deepest-acting, individualized treatment that does not require obsessive reapplication but is powerful enough to have a significant effect. It is interesting to surmise how this might be done in a sophisticated psychotherapy, both with and without actual homeopathic remedies. Ultimately, when homeopathy's law of similars is more fully understood and utilized, psychologists and psychiatrists will automatically recognize symptoms as the organism's adaptive responses and will seek to aid patients in efforts to go with, rather than against, this self-defensive, self-healing process.

---

*See Catherine Coulter, *Portraits of Homoeopathic Medicines: Psychophysical Analyses of Selected Constitutional Types* (Berkeley: North Atlantic Books, 1986); and Edward C. Whitmont, *Psyche and Substance: Essays on Homeopathy in the Light of Jungian Psychology* (Berkeley: North Atlantic Books, 1981).

Notes

1. Charles Frederick Menninger, "Some Reflections Relative to the Symptomatology and Materia Medica of Typhoid Fever," *Transactions of the American Institute of Homoeopathy,* 1897, p. 430.

2. Jonas Robitscher, *The Power of Psychiatry* (Boston: Houghton Mifflin, 1980), p. 282.

3. Jerrold S. Maxmen, *The New Psychiatry* (New York: William Morrow, 1985), p. 42.

4. Ibid., p. 58.

5. Ibid., p. 112.

6. Paul H. Wender and Donald F. Klein, *Mind, Mood, and Medicine* (New York: New American Library, 1982), p. 345.

7. Ibid., p. 197.

8. Maxmen, *The New Psychiatry,* p. 158.

9. Menninger, "Some Reflections," p. 430.

10. Edward C. Whitmont, *Psyche and Substance: Essays on Homeopathy in the Light of Jungian Psychology* (Berkeley: North Atlantic Books, 1981).

11. Catherine Coulter, *Portraits of Homoeopathic Medicines: Psychophysical Analyses of Selected Constitutional Types* (Berkeley: North Atlantic Books, 1986).

12. George Vithoulkas and Bill Gray, "Nux Vomica," *Journal of Homeopathic Practice,* 1 (Spring 1978): 36–42; Vithoulkas and Gray, "Arsenicum Album," *Journal of Homeopathic Practice,* 1 (Spring 1978): 43–50. Select medicines are also discussed in Vithoulkas, *Homeopathy: Medicine of the New Man* (New York: Arco, 1979).

13. There are many good materia medicas, including M. Tyler, *Drug Pictures* (Essex, England: Health Science, 1942); C. E. Wheeler, *An Introduction to the Principles and Practice of Homoeopathy* (Essex, England: Health Sciences, 1948); J. T. Kent, *Lectures on Homoeopathic Materia Medica* (New Delhi: B. Jain, n.d.); and D. M. Gibson, *Studies of Homoeopathic Remedies* (Beaconsfield, England: Beaconsfield, 1987). For other materia medicas, see "Homeopathic Resources" in Part III.

14. Theodor Adorno, *The Authoritarian Personality* (New York: Harper and Row, 1950).

15. Jack Cooper, "The Treatment and Cure of Alcoholism and Related Illnesses on an Outpatient Basis with Homeopathy," *Journal of the American Institute of Homeopathy,* 75 (June 1982): 18–21. J. P.

Gallavardin, a French homeopath in the 1800s, experienced a similar 50 percent cure rate of alcoholism with the use of homeopathic medicine. For further information, see J. P. Gallavardin, *How to Cure Alcoholism: The Non-toxic Homoeopathic Way* (Katonah, N.Y.: East-West Arts, 1976).

16. Seldon H. Talcott, "The Curability of Mental and Nervous Diseases Under Homoeopathic Medication," *Transactions of the American Institute of Homoeopathy*, 1891, pp. 875–886.

17. Ellen L. Keith, "Progress of the Year in Regard to State Hospital Work," *Transactions of the American Institute of Homoeopathy*, 1899, pp. 566–568.

18. D. M. Gibson and B. S. Lond, "Some Observations on Homoeopathy in Relation to Psychoneuroses, *British Homoeopathic Journal*, 43 (1953).

19. V. E. Frankl, "Paradoxical Intention: A Logotherapeutic Technique," *American Journal of Psychotherapy*, 14 (1960): 520–535; Frankl, "Paradoxical Intention and Dereflection: A Logotherapeutic Technique," *Psychotherapy: Theory, Research, and Practice*, 12 (1975): 226–237.

20. G. Bateson, D. D. Jackson, J. Haley, and J. Weakland, "Toward a Theory of Schizophrenia," in G. Bateson, *Steps to an Ecology of Mind* (New York: Ballantine, 1972); Jay Haley, *Problem-solving Therapy: New Strategies for Effective Family Therapy* (New York: Harper and Row, 1976); P. Watzlawick, J. Weakland, and R. Fisch, eds., *Change: Principles of Problem Formation and Problem Resolution* (New York: Norton, 1974).

21. Jay Haley, *Uncommon Therapy: The Psychiatric Techniques of Milton H. Erickson* (New York: Norton, 1973).

Additional References

Riebel, Linda. "A Homeopathic Model of Psychotherapy." *Journal of Humanistic Psychology*, 24 (Winter 1984): 9–48.

Slonim, Daphna, and Kerrin White. "Homeopathy and Psychiatry." *Journal of Mind and Behavior*, 4 (Summer 1983): 401–410.

12

Homeopathy and Dentistry: Keeps You Smiling

Portraits of our country's first president, George Washington, rarely show him smiling—and for a good reason: his dentures were made of wood. Though they were well sculpted by his blacksmith friend Paul Revere, this crude set of teeth did not have the same polish as nature's artistry.

Dentistry has come a long way since the time of George Washington, but it still has a long way to go in order to deal with the degree of dental problems affecting people today.

It has been estimated that 98 percent of the American public suffer from dental disease.[1] Approximately twenty-five million Americans, or one in every eight people, do not have any teeth at all.[2] And over six million teeth are extracted each year.[3]

One may wonder what homeopathic medicine may offer dentistry. Initially it may seem that dental disease is a straightforward problem that simply requires good hygiene for prevention and the use of modern dental practices to deal with dental problems as they arise. Dentistry is apparently not a controversial subject. Or is it? Although there may be general agreement on the importance of prevention, there is disagreement on *how* to prevent dental problems, and there is significant controversy over how to deal with these problems when they arise.

It is generally recognized that tooth decay (caries) results from bacteria in the mouth which thrive on the sugar and refined foods that the person eats. The bacteria produce a harmful acid that can dissolve teeth. When the teeth are not kept clean through brushing and flossing, the germs are able to infiltrate through the enamel and into the dentine of the teeth or under the gums of the mouth, wreaking havoc by causing decay and peridontal disease.

When the bacteria are not cleaned out of the mouth, they bind with corrosive waste products in the mouth and attach themselves to teeth and gums, forming plaque. Plaque destroys the connective tissues that attach gums to teeth, creating inflammation of the gums, or gingivitis. If this disease process continues, the teeth will loosen and eventually either fall out or need to be removed.

Dental caries and gum problems are thought to result primarily from poor care and maintenance of the oral cavity. There are, however, other factors that influence the development of caries. It is recognized that the salivary glands in the mouth help to fight decay by neutralizing the acid that the germs produce. The healthy functioning of the salivary glands are dependent on the person's overall health.

One's overall health also directly affects gum health. Hormones, in particular, play a major role in the health of gums. If a person's thyroid gland is secreting either too much or too little thyroid hormone, the ligaments that hold teeth and gums together are weakened and the blood supply to gum tissues is decreased. Imbalance in sex hormones can make a person more susceptible to gum and teeth problems, which is why women experience exacerbated dental conditions during puberty, menstruation, pregnancy, and menopause. Anemia, which can lessen the amount of blood oxygen reaching the gums, can also make a person more susceptible to gum disease. Even something as general as stress can influence the strength of the connective tissues between teeth and gums.

A person's overall health also influences the strength of his or her teeth. The parathyroid regulates calcium levels in the body, and an irregularity in this gland can create various dental problems.

One's overall health is affected by proper nutrition, and dental health is certainly influenced by it, too. In particular, dentists have found that appropriate amounts of calcium and fluoride are important for dental health. There is, however, a major controversy over how much fluoride is necessary and how people should get it.

Homeopathic Insights on the Controversy of Fluoridation

The American Dental Association (ADA) asserts that water fluoridation decreases dental caries by 50 to 70 percent.[4] Opponents of fluoridation question its value in preventing these dental problems and cite dozens of studies that show the toxic effects of fluoridation. Who is right?

The homeopathic point of view on fluoride is that it may be helpful in preventing caries *and* it may cause various other dental and health problems. The basic homeopathic principle is that a substance in microdose will help to cure the very symptoms that it will cause in larger doses. Fluoride is an effective medicine in preventing caries, but it can also mottle teeth (turn them chalky white or yellow) and cause various other symptoms.

The essential question, then, is: what is the proper dose to prevent caries, and what is the toxic dose? This question is more difficult than it seems. People have varying needs, and what may be helpful to one person may be harmful to another. A 1982 article in *Science* noted that the one part per million of fluoride that is commonly added to water may be too much after all.[5] The author noted that 28 percent of children between eleven and thirteen years of age who lived in communities with fluoridation experienced mottling of the teeth.

As an enzyme poison, fluoride may in fact help to reduce the formation of bacterial acid in the mouth that corrodes teeth. However, even in the same dose, fluoride may create various symptoms because of its side effects on bodily enzymes that are beneficial for health. A new study reported in the *New Scientist* has provided strong evidence that "fluoride switches off the enzyme by attacking its weakest links—the delicately-balanced network of hydrogen bonds surrounding the enzyme's active site."[6] The researchers theorize that fluoride may interfere with the hydrogen bonding of DNA in the same way that it interferes with certain enzymes, which may then explain how fluoride can cause a wide variety of symptoms and syndromes.

Anti-fluoridationists readily acknowledge that dental caries declined significantly when fluoridation was first tested. However, they also cite the fact that dental caries declined for people in unfluoridated cities as well.[7]

According to the National Academy of Sciences, fluoride is not considered an essential nutrient.[8] A deficiency of fluoride is extremely unusual for persons eating a standard American diet. Whereas the American Dental Association asserts that fluoridation assures that people will get amounts of fluoride that will prevent caries, anti-fluoridationists counter that we are already getting enough, perhaps even too much. The anti-fluoridationists have expressed concern that additional fluoride in the diet will cause a wide variety of serious health problems. It has been estimated that food prepared with fluoridated water—for example, some dried cereals, ready-to-drink fruit juices, infant formula, and strained baby food—contain up to twenty times as much fluoride as products made with unfluoridated water.[9]

Those who oppose fluoride have been portrayed as wild-eyed crazy, health nuts who see communist conspiracies in everything. This accusation has no basis in fact, especially when one considers that most countries in Europe have not fluoridated their water, including France, West Germany, Italy, Spain, Switzerland, Sweden, Holland, Denmark, Austria, and Belgium.

Furthermore, recent scientific research has begun to verify several of the health concerns of the anti-fluoridationists. Dr. John Yiamouyiannis, a biochemist who is one of the leaders of the anti-fluoridation movement, noted that the mottling of teeth is "merely a reflection of the metabolic disturbances of soft tissue cells" from an overdose of fluoride.[10] The *1983 Physicians' Desk Reference* has noted that half a milligram of fluoride, an amount equal to only one pint of fluoridated water, can cause skin problems, gastric distress, headaches, and weakness in hypersensitive individuals. Yale professor Dr. J. A. Albright reported that as little as one part per million of fluoride decreases bone strength and elasticity.[11] A study published in the *Journal of Dental Research* showed that one part per million of fluoride fed to animals inhibited their immune system.[12]

Research has also shown that levels of one-half to one part per million of fluoride cause increased tumor growth in mice by 15 to 25 percent.[13] Based on this research, one might expect that persons who live in cities with fluoridated water will have a higher cancer rate than those who live in unfluoridated cities. Dr. Yiamouyiannis, in conjunction with the former chief chemist at the National Cancer Institute, Dr. Dean Burk, made this comparison and found that people living in fluoridated cities did, in fact, have higher cancer death rates than those in unfluoridated cities in surrounding geographical areas.[14] However, a careful analysis of these statistics that was published in the *New England Journal of Medicine* noted that this study was not age-adjusted research.* This critique of the Yiamouyiannis and Burk study indicates that there is no *proven* link between fluoridation and cancer.[15]

Although there may not be definite evidence that fluoridation leads to cancer, many clinicians have found that it can cause diarrhea, muscular pains, excessive thirst and urination, episodes of acute abdominal pain, skin rashes, and progressive exhaustion. George Waldbott, M.D., a practicing allergist for over fifty years and the author of *Fluoridation: The Great Dilemma*, has noted that many physicians misdiagnose this sensitivity as "nerves" and then prescribe drugs that ultimately exacerbate the problem.[16]

In addition to the potential problems that fluoride in water supplies may cause, new research published in the highly respected scientific journal *Nature* has found that using fluorided water in aluminum pots tends to leech significantly more aluminum into the food than does unfluoridated water.[17] Since ingestion of aluminum has been linked to Alzheimer's disease, it may be prudent to avoid aluminum cookware, especially if one uses fluoridated water.

Although homeopathic organizations do not have a formal position on fluoridation, there is general agreement in the homeo-

---

*Age-adjusted research is a means of comparing populations based on similar age groups. Without this adjustment, certain cities with elderly populations would seem to have significantly higher death rates than other cities, which is just what happened in the Yiamouyiannis-Burk study.

pathic community that certain individuals will be hypersensitive to fluoride. The American Dental Association acknowledges that this hypersensitivity occurs in a very small number of Americans, but homeopaths generally assume that there are greater numbers than those assumed by the ADA. There is also concern among homeopaths about what long-term exposure to small doses of fluoride may cause.

There is further concern among some homeopaths that fluoridation amounts to forced medication. Even people who get bottled water will ingest some fluoride as a result of increased fluoride in the food chain from watering fruits and vegetables, from washing fruits or vegetables in tap water, and from feeding fluoridated water to animals that will be consumed. Ralph Nader expressed a similar concern when he stated in 1974 that "fluoridation has been promoted without giving consumers their free choice."[18]

Some anti-fluoridationists have flippantly advocated that we "fluoridate candy, not water." Perhaps even this is not a good idea.

Amalgam Fillings: The Controversy

In 1840, the American Society of Dental Surgeons (ASDS) was formed, becoming America's first medical licensing body. This organization required that its members sign an oath affirming that they would not use mercury-containing materials in their dental fillings. The ADSD, however, went out of existence a couple of decades later, by which time its rival organization, the American Dental Association, was advocating amalgam fillings. Nevertheless, throughout the ADA's history, some dentists have questioned the safety of these fillings.

Today, a small but growing group of ADA dentists are again expressing concern about amalgams. Amalgam fillings are primarily composed of mercury, silver, tin, and copper. The anti-amalgam dentists assert that the oral cavity is the only place in the human body where we commonly place nonbiological materials. These dentists also note that the upper teeth are less than ten centimeters away from the brain and that high concentrations of mercury found post-mortem in brains have been correlated with the numbers and surface sizes of amalgam fillings.[19] The dentists express further concern that we have never adequately tested the biocompatibility of these metals. It is ironic, they note, that public health officials require dentists to keep their mercury in an airtight container and not to throw their excess mercury away in the trash but to dispose of it in a carefully determined fashion, and yet dentists readily place this toxic substance in people's mouths. In fact, over 85 percent of the American public have amalgam fillings in their mouths.

Joe Graedon, a respected pharmacologist and author of *The People's Pharmacy*, has expressed concern about amalgam fillings, stating: "How can the mercury get loose? Corrosion is the culprit. While a hunk of metal in your tooth looks impervious, it may be subject to corrosion. In addition to the chemical environment of your mouth, which includes a constant saliva bath which tends to dissolve tin, amalgam in contact with other metals (such as a good bridge) creates a miniature electrochemical cell which is hellbent on dissolving itself out of existence, freeing mercury in the process."[20]

Until very recently, the ADA has rebutted the anti-amalgam dentists, noting that there is no evidence that the amalgams release any mercury or other metals into the body. New technology, however, has been able to detect this leeching. Studies have shown that people with amalgam fillings have detectable levels of mercury vapors in their breath.[21] The ADA responded to this research by stating that mercury vapors in the mouth do not prove the presence of increased mercury in the blood. Newer studies have shown, however, that blood mercury concentrations in patients with amalgam fillings were significantly higher than for persons without such fillings.[22] Although it is not yet conclusive what symptoms this leeching may cause, some research has shown that people with amalgam fillings have a significant decrease in numbers of T-cells* after insertion of fillings, compared to T-cell levels before insertion or after removal of the fillings.[23]

Nevertheless, contrary to those who have asserted that amalgam fillings release toxic amounts of metals into the body, *The Medical Forum*, a respected medical newsletter, has expressed

---

*T-cells are important components of the immune system.

doubt that the mercury leeching causes any medical problems, except in a very small number of people allergic to the amalgam.[24] *The Medical Forum*, however, did not address the concerns of acupuncturists and others familiar with Chinese medicine who do not simply worry about toxic exposure but also about how the fillings affect acupuncture points under the teeth. Acupuncturists note that the metallic fillings have the potential of acting as batteries and capacitors that can generate current and store electrical charges. Since every tooth is situated on an acupuncture meridian, a filling may provide additional stress that may create acute and/or chronic symptoms in susceptible individuals.

The fact that acupuncture points reside under the teeth may be one possible explanation for homeopaths' observation that homeopathic medicines sometimes appear to be antidoted by some dental work, including cleanings and new fillings. It has been conjectured that some dental work stimulates so many acupuncture points in a short period of time that it may "short-circuit" the action of the homeopathic medicines. More research on this phenomenon would certainly be worthwhile.

Although most homeopaths are unfamiliar with the controversies surrounding amalgam fillings, there have always been certain ones who have noted the health effects of these fillings. As far back as the late 1800s, Dr. Charles Taft, professor of dental surgery at a homeopathic medical college in Chicago, claimed that amalgam fillings were responsible for the fact that some patients with chronic disease were not responding to homeopathic medicines. Once these fillings were removed, he found that the medicines worked and the person's chronic condition disappeared or was significantly reduced.[25]

As with fluoridation, homeopaths find that some people are more sensitive than others to certain metals. Since dentists generally recognize this fact also, the most practical way to deal with it is for dentists to test the biocompatibility of various types of fillings before placing them in a person's mouth. Certain recognized immunological tests can be found, though they are expensive. Some dentists have found that new electroacupuncture machines are able to assess subtle but measurable changes in the meridian energy that acupuncturists feel can determine hypersensitivity.[26] Although this new technology may hold promise, its accuracy is presently undetermined.

Homeopaths are also concerned about the long-term exposure to metals in the fillings. Some homeopaths have found that potentized doses of *Mercury* have helped some people, but most homeopaths recognize the importance of strict individualization of doses in order to provide help to people suffering from their fillings. Homeopaths have also observed, as did homeopathic dentist Taft, that fillings sometimes have to be removed before improvement in health is possible.

Homeopathic Medicines for Dental Problems

"For there was never yet a philosopher that could endure the toothache patiently," wrote Shakespeare in *Much Ado About Nothing*. Besides offering a different perspective on fluoridation and amalgam fillings, homeopathy also offers specific medicines that can be invaluable in reducing dental pain and alleviating dental disease.

It should first be mentioned, however, that homeopathic medicines do not replace good dental care but complement it. Also, the medicines may be effective in relieving dental pain, but it is often necessary to discover what the source of the pain is in order to cure the underlying problem. If pain is occurring because of an abscess, it is not enough simply to reduce the pain. The abscess must be treated.

One dental problem that homeopaths report treating effectively is fear, anxiety, and anticipation of the dental visit. Whether these emotions are "rational" or not, homeopaths have found three medicines to be highly effective. *Aconite* (monkshood) is a medicine commonly given to patients, usually children, for their fear of dentists. These people become furious, restless, and angry (children will often stamp their feet and kick), and tend to express extreme sensitivity to touch. *Gelsemium* (yellow jasmine) is indicated for those people who experience trepidation, feelings of weakness (especially in the stomach), drowsiness, loss of memory, and diarrhea. Those who need *Gelsemium* tend to be hypokinetic, whereas those who need *Argenticum nitricum* (silver nitrate) tend to be hyperkinetic. *Argenticum nitricum* is useful for patients who experience tremor and trembling of the whole body, who tend to be particularly talkative and hurried in their actions, and who have an inner nervousness that affects the bladder and intestines.

In order to determine the appropriate homeopathic medicine for toothaches, it is helpful to learn what the source of the problem is. If it is the result of a dental abscess, the common medicines are *Belladonna* (deadly nightshade), *Mercurius* (mercury), *Hepar sulph* (Hahnemann's calcium sulphide), and *Silica* (silica). *Belladonna* is indicated at the initial formative stages when there is not much swelling, though there is much throbbing and redness. *Mercurius* is helpful when the person is salivating excessively, has foul breath, and experiences a pulsating pain that tends to be worse at night or from exposure to anything extremely hot or cold. *Hepar sulph* is valuable in the later stages of abscess when pus has formed. The tooth affected is hypersensitive to touch and to cold, and the gums bleed easily. Homeopaths have reported that this medicine helps to drain pus from the abscess. *Silica* is indicated after the pus has discharged; at this stage, it hastens the resolution of the abscess.

Although these medicines may be helpful in alleviating the pain and in some instances in curing the condition, it is usually necessary for the abscess to be drained either by performing a root canal procedure or extracting the tooth.

For pain and inflammation around wisdom teeth, homeopaths and dentists have found that *Belladonna* is often helpful for throbbing pains and *Hepar sulph* for promoting expulsion of pus. *Mercurius* is helpful in treating pulsating pains that extend to the ears, especially at night. People who need *Mercurius* also tend to have noticeably increased salivation. Locally, mouthwashes with tincture of *Salvia* (sage) are sometimes helpful.

Neuralgic toothaches often yield to *Chamomilla* when the person is in such pain that he cannot take it anymore. People who need *Chamomilla* tend to be particularly sensitive to warm food and drink (especially coffee), and their symptoms are worse at night. For persons who are so frantic with pain that they cannot sleep, whose pains are also relieved by holding cold water or ice in the mouth, and who are not relieved by *Chamomilla, Coffea* is indicated. *Plantago* (plantain) is one of the more common medicines indicated when there is a toothache with radiating pains to the ears. These pains are frequently accompanied by salivation, facial neuralgia, and headache. Homeopaths usually use the tincture form or low potencies for the best results. Another medicine (aside from *Plantago* and *Mercurius*) that homeopaths consider when dental pain extends to the ears is *Sulphur*. The prescription of either *Sulphur* or *Mercurius*, however, is determined by the totality of the person's symptoms, and these medicines are never given in tincture form.

Hypericum (St. John's wort—the herb) is the most common medicine given to people for neuralgic pains after tooth extractions. Recent double-blind research has confirmed its effectiveness.[27] This study showed that when *Hypericum* was given in alternation with *Arnica* (mountain daisy) after tooth extraction, the patients experienced significantly less dental pain than those given a placebo.

Dr. George Baldwin (a dentist in Oakland, California), Dr. Philip Parsons (a dentist in Keystone Heights, Florida), and Dr. Richard Fischer (a dentist in Annandale, Virginia), have all reported impressive results using *Ruta* (rue) for people who have pain after dental surgery. *Ruta* is known in homeopathy as a great medicine for injuries to the bone and periosteum, the bone covering (see Chapter 10 on Sports Medicine for more detail). Since teeth are actually considered by anatomists to be joints,* it is certainly understandable that *Ruta* would be useful for traumas or injuries to them.

Homeopaths have also reported success in treating hemorrhage after extraction, surgery, or accidental dental trauma. Some homeopaths give *Arnica* to prevent hemorrhage or in the very initial stages of bleeding. If bleeding persists and is bright red, *Phosphorus* is commonly effective. In the rare instances when *Phosphorus* does not act rapidly, *Ipecacuanha* (ipecac) is often indicated. *Lachesis* (venom of the bushmaster snake) is valuable if the blood

---

*Specifically, teeth are classified as ball-and-socket joints.

is dark. If a person has chronic bleeding problems, it is recommended that he receive constitutional homeopathic care.

If a puncture wound in the gum incurred from surgery is causing pain, *Ledum* (marsh tea) can relieve the pain and help it to heal. If infection has already set in, *Pyrogen* (artificial sepsin) is indicated. *Calendula* (marigolds) in its tincture form is also helpful in conjunction with either of these medicines.

The tincture of *Calendula* is not only useful in speeding the healing of punctures but is also valuable in healing the trauma from injuries to the oral cavity. It is especially useful for children whose braces irritate their gums or mouth and for elderly persons whose dentures do not fit well. (Ultimately, getting the braces or dentures properly adjusted may also be necessary.) Burns from ingesting extremely hot food or drinks or from aspirin are alleviated by *Calendula* tincture as well. If the tincture is not readily available, making a tea of marigolds is equally effective.

A "dry socket" is the source of many people's dental pain. This condition occurs after an extraction when the blood does not clot well, and the bone and its nerve endings are exposed. Mouthwashes of *Salvia* (sage) infusions several times a day diminish some of the pain.* Other medicines for this pain are: *Belladonna* for redness around the gums and throbbing pains that come and go rapidly; *Coffea* for unbearable pains that cause the person to be very restless and that are temporarily relieved by cold water or ice in the mouth; *Hepar sulph* for pain that is hypersensitive to touch and to cold; and *Silica* for help in the final stages when the clot around the tooth ultimately needs to be detached. If none of the above medicines seems indicated or is working, *Ruta* should be given.

A dental problem that has only recently become widely recognized is temporomandibular joint (TMJ) syndrome.[28] The analysis of this condition has linked various dental and other health problems to the malalignment of the jaw joint (the temporomandibular joint). It has been estimated that 38 percent of all nerve impulses

---

*An infusion is made by steeping an herb in hot but not boiling water in order to extract the soluble constituents.

that go to the brain pass near this joint area. Malalignment of the jaw has been found to lead to symptoms as diverse as headache, vertigo, ringing in the ears, sinus pains, hearing loss, depression, and tic douloureux. Dr. Harold Gelb, director of the TMJ Clinic at the New York Eye and Ear Infirmary, has estimated that twenty million Americans suffer from TMJ syndrome.[29] Some dentists have estimated that 50 percent of all headaches are traceable to this syndrome.[30]

Because of the diversity of symptoms that TMJ syndrome sufferers experience, there are many medicines that homeopaths consider in determining proper treatment. As with any other chronic malady, the homeopathic approach requires an assessment of the person's totality of symptoms. Care from a professional homeopath is clearly indicated in such cases.

Besides treating acute dental problems, homeopathic medicines have the capacity to treat various chronic dental problems as well. Since some chronic dental conditions result from general health problems, homeopathic medicines that have the capacity to strengthen a person's overall health can augment general dental hygiene in the prevention and treatment of teeth and gum disease.

The proper functioning of the salivary glands enables the body to digest foods and to neutralize the acids that germs in the mouth produce. Healthy functioning of the endocrine system helps the ligaments that hold teeth to gums remain strong and aids the transport of blood to gums. The parathyroid gland is instrumental in helping to regulate calcium levels in the body. Because overall functioning of the body plays an integral role in dental health, homeopathy will inevitably be recognized as a necessary part of general health care as well as good dental health.

It is certainly encouraging that more and more dentists are utilizing homeopathic medicines. For those whose dentists have not yet made the transition to homeopathy, laypersons can learn to use the medicines themselves with impressive success. In order to obtain the best results, the reader is urged to obtain several books—not just books on homeopathy and dentistry, but also some of the materia medicas in order to learn more about the medicines.* And, when possible, the reader is urged to attend seminars on homeopathic dentistry.

Homeopathy *can* help keep you smiling!

Notes

1. Melvin Denholz and Elaine Denholtz, *How to Save Your Teeth and Your Money* (New York: Van Nostrand Reinhold, 1977), p. 12.

2. Thomas McGuire, *The Tooth Trip* (New York: Random House, 1972), p. 2.

3. Denholz and Denholz, *Save Your Teeth*, p. 12.

4. J. H. Shaw, *Fluoridation as a Public Health Measure* (Washington, D.C.: American Association for the Advancement of Science, 1954); J. J. Murray, *Fluorides in Caries Prevention* (Bristol, England: Wright, 1976); E. Newbrun, ed., *Fluorides and Dental Caries*, 2nd ed. (Springfield, Ill.: Thomas, 1975).

5. Dennis H. Leverett, "Fluorides and the Changing Prevalence of Dental Caries," *Science*, 217 (July 2, 1982): 26–30.

6. "How Fluoride Might Damage Your Health," *New Scientist*, February 28, 1985, p. 20.

7. Leverett, "Fluorides," p. 29.

8. "Is Fluoride an Essential Element?" in *Fluorides* (Washington, D.C.: National Academy of Sciences, 1971), pp. 66–68. Also see Richard Maurer and Harry Day, "The Non-Essentiality of Fluorine in Nutrition," *Journal of Nutrition*, 62 (1957): 561–573.

9. Ellen Ruppel Shell, "The New Flap Over Fluoride," *American Health*, October 1984, pp. 60–63.

10. John Yiamouyiannis, *Fluoride: The Aging Factor* (Delaware, Ohio: Health Action, 1983), p. 172.

11. J. A. Albright, "The Effect of Fluoride on the Mechanical Properties of Bone," *Transactions of the Annual Meeting of the Orthopedics Research Society*, 98 (1978): 3.

12. D. W. Allmann and M. Benac, "Effect of Inorganic Fluoride Salts on Urine and Tissue 3'5' Cyclic-AMP Concentration in Vivo," *Journal of Dental Research*, 55, supplement B (1976): 523.

---

*See the "Homeopathic Resources" section in Part III for details on accessing books.

13. Alfred Taylor and Nell Carmichael Taylor, "Effect of Sodium Fluoride on Tumor Growth," *Proceedings of the Society for Experimental Biology and Medicine*, 119 (1965): 252–255.

14. John Yiamouyiannis and Dean Burk, "Fluoridation and Cancer: Age Dependence of Cancer Mortality Related to Artificial Fluoridation," *Fluoride*, 10 (1977): 102–123.

15. J. David Erickson, "Mortality in Selected Cities with Fluoridated and Non-Fluoridated Water Supplies," *New England Journal of Medicine*, 298 (May 18, 1978): 1112–16.

16. George L. Waldbott with A. W. Burgstahler and H. L. McKinney, *Fluoridation: The Great Dilemma* (Lawrence, Kans.: Coronado Press, 1978).

17. Quoted in Dr. Dean Edell's "Medical Journal," *San Francisco Chronicle*, April 29, 1987.

18. Quoted in Yiamouyiannis, *Fluoride*, p. 118.

19. Patrick Stortebecker, *Mercury Poisoning from Dental Amalgams* (Orlando, Fla.: Bio-probe, 1986).

20. Joe Graedon, "Dental Dangers," *San Francisco Chronicle*, January 11, 1984.

21. C. W. Svare, L. C. Peterson, J. W. Reinhardt, et al., "The Effect of Dental Amalgams on Mercury Levels in Expired Air," *Journal of Dental Research*, 60 (1981): 1668–71.

22. J. E. Abraham, C. W. Svare, and C. W. Frank, "The Effect of Dental Amalgam Restorations on Blood Mercury Levels," *Journal of Dental Research*, 63 (1984): 71–73.

23. D. W. Eggleston, "Effect of Dental Amalgam and Nickel Alloys on T-lymphocytes: Preliminary Report," *Journal of Prosthetic Dentistry*, May 1984, pp. 617–623.

24. "Mercury in Dental Fillings: Is There a Problem?" *The Medical Forum*, November 1985, pp. 5–7.

25. Charles Taft, "Injurious Effects of Amalgam Fillings," *Medical Advance*, 30 (June 1893): 422–430.

26. R. Voll, "Twenty Years of Electroacupuncture Diagnosis," *American Journal of Acupuncture*, (March 1975): 7–17; R. Voll, "Electroacupuncture (EAV) Diagnostics and Treatment Results in Odontogenous Focal Events," *American Journal of Acupuncture*, 9 (December 1981): 293–302.

27. Henri Albertini, William Goldberg, Bernard Sanguy, and Claude Toulza, "Homeopathic Treatment of Dental Neuralgia Using Arnica and Hypericum: A Summary of 60 Observations," *Journal of the American Institute of Homeopathy*, 78 (September 1985): 126–128.

28. Denholz and Denholz, *Save Your Teeth;* Irwin Smigel, *Dental Health, Dental Beauty* (New York: M. Evans, 1979).

29. Denholz and Denholz, *Save Your Teeth*, p. 42.

30. Smigel, *Dental Health*, p. 236.

Additional References

Fischer, Richard D. "Dentistry and Homeopathy: An Overview." *Journal of the American Institute of Homeopathy*, 78 (December 1985): 140–147.

Lessell, Colin B. *The Dental Prescriber*. London: British Homoeopathic Association.

Steinlechner, F. "Homoeopathy in Dentistry." *British Homoeopathic Journal*, 73 (July 1984): 145–149.

Ziff, Sam. *The Toxic Time Bomb: Can the Mercury in Your Dental Fillings Poison You?* New York: Aurora, 1984.

The Newest References

Hileman, Bette. "Fluoridation of Water," *Chemical and Engineering News,* August 1, 1988.

National Toxicology Program, Report 393, National Institutes of Health Publication No. 90–2848, 1989.

Vimy, J. J., Takhashi, Y., and Lorscheider, F. L., "Maternal-fetal Distribution of Mercury Released from Dental Amalgam Fillings," *American Journal of Physiology*, 1990: 258:R939–45.

13

Collaborative Health Care:
A Model for the 21st Century

The American Council of Life Insurance is not a radical group of visionaries. It is, in fact, a conservative group of businesspeople who recently completed a series of reports on health care in the year 2030. One of the Council's scenarios for the future predicted: "Osteopaths, acupuncturists, massage therapists, ethnic healers, and allopathically trained diagnosticians [conventional physicians] will have equal status—and roughly equal earnings."[1]

Some people might consider this prediction quite radical. However, based on the evidence that this book has provided about the logic and effectiveness of homeopathic medicines, it is reasonable to assume that the significant changes predicted by the Council will probably come considerably earlier than projected.

The revolution in medicine is already taking place. The number of alternative birth centers in hospitals has grown astronomically in the past fifteen years. Hospices have gained broad support from the hospitals, federal agencies, and various charitable medical organizations, including the American Cancer Society. There is more interest in nutrition and fitness than ever before, and this interest does not seem to be simply faddish, but represents a significant change in lifestyle. Just fifteen years ago, biofeedback was considered a part of "alternative medicine," but now it is an integral part of the care provided by many physicians and psychologists, as well as being offered at hospitals. Relaxation and visualization exercises are not simply pastimes for idle moments when one has nothing better to do, but are becoming consciously planned activities that provide their own health benefits. Acupuncture is not just gaining wider credibility from the public, but is being practiced by a growing number of various health professionals. And finally, homeopathic medicine, as this book has clearly shown, is gaining respect and popularity throughout the world.

"Alternative health care" is becoming a misnomer. Because of this, Prince Charles and several leading English physicians and health professionals are popularizing the concept of "complementary medicine," a concept that has been described in at least two ways: as a synonym and as a better word for alternative health care and as an approach that takes the best from conventional medicine and the best from alternative health care. Several major organizations, such as the Research Council for Complementary Medicine and the Institute for Complementary Medicine, have already been established in England, have begun publishing professional journals, and have sponsored university research on complementary therapies.

As much as there is a need for organizations that seek to legitimize complementary therapies, there is also a need for efforts to assess how complementary and conventional therapies might be integrated together in the provision of health care. As one attempts to ascertain how this integration might occur, it is essential to avoid Pollyannaish daydreams of a perfect health care system.

The integration of complementary and conventional therapies would not necessarily mean that they would be used at the same time on a patient. Rather, there will be times when only conventional methods are indicated and other times when only complementary therapies are needed. The decisions on when to use each will sometimes be easy and obvious and sometimes exceedingly difficult. Some health problems, for instance, may suggest the use of powerful conventional medications that may significantly reduce a painful condition but that may also seriously compromise the person's immune system as a by-product of providing this relief. Because many of the complementary therapies tend to work by stimulating immune and defense responses, these therapies may counteract the workings of the drug. In such instances, the patient must weigh the risks and benefits of utilizing the conventional drug, as compared with the risks and benefits of using some of the complementary therapies.

Determining who should make the decision for infants and children will probably be a major ethical issue in the coming decades. Determining if a physician has adequately and accurately informed a patient of the risks and benefits of the various therapies will also be a difficult and complicated ethical issue. And, as it is today, determining when a person is and is not mentally competent to make decisions that affect his or her own health will continue to be a major ethical issue in the 21st century.

Despite the difficulties in creating a comprehensive health care system that integrates conventional and complementary therapies, it seems obvious that the benefits offered by this "collaborative model of health care" significantly outweigh its inevitable problems. Such a model of health care will:

- Provide more comprehensive health care to people.
- Offer more individualized care to fulfill the varied health care needs of a diverse population.
- Provide noninvasive therapeutic measures that stimulate immune and defense responses, resorting to heroic measures only when necessary, thus leading to considerably fewer iatrogenic (doctor-induced) diseases.
- Utilize a variety of health care professionals who work together for the benefit of the patient.
- Encourage sick persons to play a more active role in their own health. This will not only become an economic necessity but will also be recognized as an integral way to provide effective health care.

Towards a New Science of Medicine

Lewis Thomas, the head of the Sloan-Kettering Cancer Center, has asserted that one of the major problems with medicine today is that it is not scientific enough.[2] The fact that a report from the U.S. Congress's Office of Technology Assessment acknowledged that only 10 to 20 percent of medical procedures have been proven effective by controlled studies reveals only one of many symptoms of the lack of scientific verification of so much of present-day medicine.[3] In addition to the lack of clinical evidence for most medical treatments, there are also gaping holes in the knowledge of how and why drugs work. Despite all the research on aspirin, for instance, we still do not understand fully why it has its effects.

In referring to the goals of science, the late Abraham Maslow, one of the founders of humanistic psychology and a scholar on the philosophy of science, said: "Before all else, science must be comprehensive and all-inclusive. . . . It must describe and accept the 'way things are,' the actual world as it is, understandable or not, meaningful or not, explainable or not."[4]

Scientists are now able to show how a specific conventional medication may act upon a specific physiological process, and a certain aura attends this new, verified knowledge. However, a significant gap in medical science remains, since there is little knowledge about how drugs affect the whole body.

There are several aspects of homeopathy that will help medicine to become more scientific than it is at present. For example, an inherent part of the homeopathic method is the drug trials called "provings," whereby a substance is tested for the symptoms of its overdose. Once it is discovered what a substance causes, it is known what it can cure when given in small, specially prepared doses. Such trials inform homeopaths about the totality of physical and psychological symptoms that a substance will cure. These experiments help homeopathy to develop itself as a medical science that Maslow would have considered "comprehensive and all-inclusive."

Admittedly, homeopaths may not know the specific biochemical pathways or the physiological processes that a substance affects. However, they do know the empirical facts from the drug provings, which show the syndromes that substances cause. Homeopaths may not understand why a person has symptoms, but they can determine what medicine can be individually chosen to treat those symptoms. The homeopathic process of individualization fits what Maslow referred to as a method that "accepts the 'way things are,' the actual world as it is, understandable or not, meaningful or not, explainable or not."

Whether or not one actually understands how the homeopathic medicines work does not mean much vis-à-vis proof or disproof of the system. Inaccurate explanations of gravity do not make it disappear, and accurate explanations do not make it stronger. Likewise, inaccurate theories about how the homeopathic medicines work only discredit the explanation, not the method itself.

The homeopaths' use of Hering's Law of Cure will also help medicine to become more scientific. Hering's Law of Cure, as discussed in Chapter 1, is a comprehensive means of assessment that helps determine if a sick person is getting healthier or sicker. At present, scientific research too often narrowly measures improvement in health by primarily determining if a symptom has gotten better or worse. Hering's Law of Cure, by comparison, is a significantly more sophisticated method to assess the healing process. Hering's Law of Cure will enable researchers to move beyond limited reductionistic methodologies to more accurate holistic systems of evaluation.

Of special importance, homeopathy will help physicians and scientists to better understand the nature of healing. Because homeopaths assume that the human organism has basic inherent self-healing tendencies, they maintain a deep respect for the *vis medicatrix naturae*, more commonly known as the "healing power of nature." René Dubos, Nobel Prize–winning microbiologist, acknowledged the importance of really understanding this innate healing intelligence. In his introduction to Norman Cousins's seminal book *Anatomy of an Illness*, Dubos said: "Modern medicine will become really scientific only when physicians and their patients have learned to manage the forces of the body and the mind that operate in *vis medicatrix naturae*."[5]

Homeopathy will also offer scientific medicine a large number of new remedies. In addition to the wide range of homeopathic medicines that have been utilized for almost two hundred years, homeopathic principles will teach us a new way of using conventional drugs. Dr. Ronald Davey, physician to Her Majesty Queen Elizabeth II, suggests that conventional drugs are invaluable in his homeopathic practice, not for the purposes that most physicians apply them, but for the side effects they are known to have.

Dr. Davey notes that conventional pharmacology texts provide much information on the side effects of drugs and that this information, like information gathered from homeopathic drug provings, is reliable symptomatology on which to prescribe. Quite distinct from conventional physicians, however, Dr. Davey uses only potentized doses of these drugs.

Concluding Thoughts

Just a little more than one hundred years ago, the National Institute of Health was conceived and brought into being. Before this, there was very little systematic accumulation and analysis of health information in Western society. As homeopathy and various complementary therapies gain greater recognition, it is inevitable that the National Institute of Health will have special divisions that investigate and develop these methods. And since complementary therapies not only have the capacity to help people to regain health but also to obtain high levels of health, it is inevitable that special divisions devoted to super health and peak performance will have an important place in the National Institute of Health and in research centers the world over.

The revolution is already in progress. We all know that medicine will continue to develop its high-tech side. It is only a matter of time before it develops a "high-touch" side. To quote Robert Frost:

How many times did it thunder before Franklin took the hint?
How many apples fell on Newton's head before he took the hint?
Nature is always hinting at us.
It hints over and over again.
And someday we take the hint.

Are you listening?

Notes

1. American Council of Life Insurance, Trend Analysis Program, *Health Care: Three Reports from 2030 A.D. (Washington, D.C., Spring 1980)*, pp. 10–11.

2. Lewis Thomas, *The Youngest Science: Notes of a Medicine Watcher* (New York: Viking, 1983).

3. Office of Technology Assessment, *Assessing the Efficacy and Safety of Medical Technologies* (Washington, D.C.: U.S. Government Printing Office, 1978), p. 7.

4. Abraham Maslow, *Towards a Psychology of Science* (Princeton: Van Nostrand, 1968).

5. René Dubos, "Introduction," in Norman Cousins, *Anatomy of an Illness* (New York: W. W. Norton, 1979), p. 23.

Appendix

Update on the Homeopathic Treatment of AIDS

"In the crime-ridden frontier town the hero, singlehanded, blasts out the desperadoes who were running rampant through the settlement. The story ends on a happy note because it appears that peace has been restored. But in reality the death of the villains does not solve the fundamental problem, for the rotten social conditions which had opened the town to the desperadoes will soon allow others to come in, unless something is done to correct the primary source of trouble. The hero moves out of town without doing anything to solve this far more complex problem; in fact, he has no weapon to deal with it, and he is not even aware of its existence."[1]

Such is a classic story told by Pulitzer Prize-winning microbiologist René Dubos as he critiqued the use of antibiotics. In his book, *The Mirage of Health*, written in 1959, Dubos showed how bacteria and viruses do not necessarily cause disease, but more accurately, often are its results. By this analogy, the criminal is not simply a problem but is the symptom of a problem. Taking this analogy further, to assume that one truly cures a person by temporarily eliminating or reducing bacterial or viral growth is like assuming that one can solve the problem of crime by killing a single criminal. Such approaches ignore the variety of factors that create an environment conducive to future bacterial or viral infection or to future criminal behavior.

Homeopathy has an impressive history of success in treating life-threatening infectious diseases. In fact, homeopathy developed its greatest popularity in the United States and Europe from its successes in treating the infectious-disease epidemics of the 1800s, including those of cholera, typhoid, yellow fever, scarlet fever, and pneumonia.[2]

Despite these excellent results, experienced, homeopathy was ignored and even attacked.

For instance, after the 1855 cholera epidemic in England, the President of the General Board of Health contacted all the metropolitan hospitals to report on their success rates. Of the 1,104 patients who received conventional medical treatment, 573 (51.9%) died. When the Board of Health presented their report, the statistics of the London Homeopathic Hospital were not included. The facts showed that only 10 deaths occurred among the 61 cases in this hospital, a mortality rate of 16.3%. When the Board of Health was queried about this omission, they replied that such statistics would "give an unjustifiable sanction to an empirical practice alike opposed to the maintenance of truth and to the progress of science."[3]

Homeopaths today commonly experience similarly good results in treating infectious diseases. For better and worse, they are not being attacked as much as they have in the past; however, they are still being ignored.

Today the Hahnemann Clinic in Berkeley, California, which has three medical doctors and three physician assistants and nurse practitioners on staff, commonly treat a hundred or so people every month with one type of infection or another. It is more common than not for these practitioners to prescribe homeopathic medicines without having to resort to antibiotics. Homeopaths, like any good medical professionals, will use antibiotics when clearly necessary, but good homeopaths rarely need to do so.

New laboratory research has also showed the beneficial effects of homeopathic medicines on the immune function. The *European Journal of Pharmacology*, for instance, published research which showed that a commonly used homeopathic medicine, *Silica*, had dramatic effects in stimulating macrophages.[4] Macrophages, a type of white blood cell that devours dead cells, are an important part of the body's defenses. *Silica 10c* was found to stimulate macrophage activity by as much as 67.5%.

New research published in the *International Journal of Immunotherapy* has shown that microdoses used in homeopathy corrected immunological disorders in New Zealand mice.[5] These same researchers also found that microdoses of interferon had immunomodulatory effects on New Zealand mice.[6]

Homeopaths commonly treat people suffering from acute and chronic viral conditions. Sometimes improvement in a person's health is immediate and dramatic after taking a homeopathic medicine, though most of the time it is slow and progressive.

Treating People with HIV+, ARC, and AIDS

Homeopathic medicines can be used effectively to treat patients in at least three ways:

1. *Prevention:* generating resistance to disease and subsequent infection;
2. *Treatment in acute illnesses:* reducing their length and severity;
3. *Restoration of health:* revitalizing the patient so that the person's overall constitution doesn't deteriorate.

This chapter primarily focuses on the professional homeopathic treatment of people with HIV+, ARC, and AIDS, rather than their self-care, because most laypeople do not have the depth of homeopathic knowledge necessary to treat this serious ailment.

Prevention

Homeopaths have found that their medicines often prevent infections. It is common for homeopaths to report that patients with AIDS or ARC seem to experience reduced recurrence and intensity of infection.

To prevent infection and to slow the progression to AIDS, homeopaths provide "homeopathic constitutional treatment," that is, the use of medicine which is individualized to the totality of the person's symptoms.

Individual homeopaths also report that people who are HIV+ do not develop AIDS or ARC very often. London homeopaths Michael Strange, Tina Head, and Melissa Assilem, whose Lavender Hill Homeopathic Centre specializes in gay health, report to having treated several hundred HIV+ patients. They estimate that 90% of their HIV+ patients have not yet developed AIDS.

Treatment of Acute Illnesses

Homeopaths report that homeopathic medicines are sometimes effective in the treatment of acute infections commonly experienced by people with AIDS or ARC. This treatment helps reduce the intake of antibiotics and other powerful drugs which have various side effects and can weaken the immune system in those people who already have immunodeficiency.

Homeopath Michael Strange has observed that his patients who get Pneumocystis carninii pneumonia (PCP) nonetheless get less severe bouts of it. He notes some of the common medicines he has used successfully in treating the acute episodes of PCP are *Bryonia* (wild hops), *China* (cinchona bark), *Pulsatilla* (windflower), *Silica.*

Strange has also noted that homeopathic medicines seem to slow or stop new Karposi's sarcoma (KS) lesions. The medicines he has used successfully include *Phosphorus, Lachesis,* and *Crotalus horridus.* Strange has also used potentized doses of cytotoxic drugs *(Vinblastin 12, Vincristin 12, Bleomycin 6)* in patients who were prescribed conventional doses of them for their KS lesions in the lungs. In the two cases in which Strange has prescribed these homeopathic doses of cytotoxic drugs he has managed to avert all side effects of the conventional drugs without interfering with the effectiveness of the treatment.[7]

Many PWAs get fungal infections. Los Angeles homeopath and acupuncturist Janet Zand has found the following medicines to be helpful in treating these conditions: *Thuja, Sulphur,* and various homeopathic nosodes (a nosode is a medicine potentized from a pathogenic tissue).

Restoration of Health

One can rarely claim that homeopathic medicines actually "cure" viral conditions since it is assumed that viruses remain in the body throughout one's life. However, homeopaths find that the health of their AIDS patients does not deteriorate as rapidly as that of patients using conventional therapies.

The homeopathic approach to treating any chronic disorder includes a thorough analysis of the person's totality of symptoms. There is thus no one medicine for a specific disease. Some homeopaths seek to find the "constitutional medicine," others use nosodes intercurrent with an individually prescribed medicine, while still others seek to find the "miasmatic medicine" (a medicine individually prescribed according to certain genetic predispositions, as defined by homeopathic theory—see pages 160–162 for a discussion on miasms).

Most homeopathic practitioners with whom I have talked about their treatment of people with AIDS have found that they need to repeat doses of medicines more often than when treating others who do not have immunodeficiency. Also, there seems to be a necessity to change prescriptions more frequently as well. The "tip-shot" method of prescribing is common: prescribing a medicine for a week, perhaps waiting a week, and then prescribing a different medicine. Although the use of low potencies is most common for patients with immunodeficiency, many practitioners will use a high potency of a miasmatic medicine, a nosode, or a constitutional medicine. When a high potency is used, several practitioners have noted the importance of more frequent repetitions of such medicines than are commonly employed with other patients.

Bill Gray, M.D. of Berkeley's Hahnemann College of Homeopathy notes that many of his patients frequently antidote their homeopathic medicine by taking recreational drugs. Even when some patients have sworn off these drugs, he reports that many of his patients return to them once they are getting better. Dr. Gray, who usually uses a single dose of a high potency, feels that frequent repetition of a homeopathic medicine is not necessary, but real changes in a person's lifestyle are essential for healing.[8]

San Francisco homeopath Dr. Laurence Badgley reported on a six month study of 36 of his patients with AIDS, ARC, or HIV+ treated with homeopathy and other natural therapies. He observed an average 13% increase in T4 helper cells and an average increase of two pound weight. He has found the following medicines to be particularly helpful in the homeopathic treatment of people with AIDS: *Typhoidinum* (typhoid nosode), *Badiaga* (fresh water sponge), and *Cyclosporin.*[9]

London homeopath Michael Strange reports having approximately 50 people with AIDS under his care. Only five of these 50 people died during 1990, and the majority of his patients with AIDS are fit and active.

Although these results do not sound miraculous, they are actually quite significant considering the serious and progressive nature of AIDS. Also, the most popular conventional drug for AIDS, AZT, according to *JAMA*,[10] has been found to prolong lives by only 7 or 8 months.

Some of the common medicines that Strange has found to be helpful are: *Arsenicum* (arsenic), *Phosphorous, Natrum mur* (salt), *Pulsatilla* (windflower), *Sepia* (cuttlefish), *Tuberculinum* (tuberculosis nosode), *Medorrhinum* (gonorrhea nosode), and *Carcinosin* (cancer nosode).[11]

Belgian homeopaths Drs. Maurice Jenaer and Bernard Marichal have recently reported on a trial conducted in Africa utilizing a combination of homeopathic medicines. In a preliminary test using 28 people with AIDS (14 men and 14 women), they observed statistically significant improvement in people with AIDS from homeopathically potentized doses of *RNA, DNA, Cyclosporin*, and a rabbit antibody called *Polypeptide Anti-Atypies*.[12]

This study showed that those patients treated with homeopathic medicines had one-half as many episodes of fever, one-half as many infections, and one-sixth as many bouts of diarrhea. The untreated patients lost an average of 22 pounds, while the treated patients actually gained 3 pounds.

Greek physician Spiro Diamantidis, who chairs the homeopathic commission for the Greek Ministry of Health and Welfare, recently reported on the treatment of 12 HIV+ patients, three of whom have AIDS, and four of whom had ARC, and five of whom were HIV+ with swollen lymph glands. These patients utilized homeopathic medicines solely, and each showed complete remission of symptoms and normalization of immune panels.[13]

Some homeopaths have found value in *Thuja* (tree of life), *Syphilinum* (syphilis nosode), various *Mercury* preparations, various *Calcarea* (calcium) preparations, *Sulphur, Lycopodium* (club moss), *Crotalus horridus* (rattlesnake), *Conium* (hemlock), and *Bromium*.

Recent research has shown that hypericin, a compound within the homeopathic medicine *Hypericum*, inhibits retroviruses in vitro and in vivo.[14] A 1989 survey reported that 80–90% of 24 AIDS patients who used it experienced some benefit. This survey also discovered that liver enzymes improved in almost every case. Though not a conventional homeopathic dose, 60–90 drops of the tincture three times a day, or 70 mg. of hypericin seem therapeutic. No side effects have been reported at these doses.[15]

In my personal discussions with homeopathic practitioners, I have learned that little progress with homeopathic medicines can be expected in the treatment of people with end-stage AIDS or with PWAs with neurological involvement. The best results come from those who are HIV+ without serious immunological problems, those with ARC, those recently diagnosed with AIDS, and patients who avoid conventional drugs. Several homeopaths have observed that progress from homeopathic medicines diminishes if the person concurrently utilizes certain powerful conventional medical treatments, specifically AZT, or if they recurrently take antibiotics. However, now that physicians are recommending lower doses of AZT, homeopaths are observing that homeopathic medicines are more able to act effectively.

Several homeopaths have also observed that it is common for people with AIDS to experience a fever after taking a homeopathic medicine. These homeopaths note that it is important that such patients do not take conventional drugs to treat this fever, or they may not experience as rapid improvement.

It can also be reported that at least one patient under homeopathic care who had tested positive to the HIV on several occasions and who had been diagnosed with AIDS is today reported to have a completely healthy immunological profile, no symptoms of illness, and no longer is HIV+. Sadly, this individual wishes to remain anonymous, and because of this, this case cannot formally be considered a "cure."

It also must be noted that no large-scale, carefully controlled research has been published which has shown the efficacy of homeopathy in treating people with AIDS or ARC. However, the research showing the antiviral action of homeopathic medicines,[15] the study proving the effectiveness of the homeopathic medicines in treating a different disease of the immune system (rheumatoid arthritis)[17] and the evidence that homeopathy was effective in treating previous major infectious diseases suggests that homeopathy may be of value in treating people with AIDS or ARC.[18]

Concluding Thoughts

There is an old Chinese saying, "If we don't change our direction, we are liable to end up where we are headed." Indeed, we need to change our direction in medicine. Homeopathic medicine will hopefully be one new direction we will be headed.

Notes

1. René Dubos, *Mirage of Health*, San Francisco: Harper and Row, 1959, 162.

2. Thomas L. Bradford, *The Logic of Figures or Comparative Results of Homoeopathic and Other Treatments*, Philadelphia: Boericke and Tafel, 1900. Harris L. Coulter, *Divided Legacy: The Conflict Between Homoeopathy and the American Medical Association*, Berkeley: North Atlantic, 1973, 302.

3. Phillip A. Nicholls, *Homoeopathy and the Medical Profession*, London: Croom Helm, 1988, 145–6.

4. Elizabeth Davenas, Bernard Poitevin, and Jacques Benveniste, "Effect on Mouse Peritoneal Macrophages of Orally Administered Very High Dilutions of Silica," *European Journal of Pharmacology* 1987; 135: 313–319.

5. M. Bastide, V. Daurat, M. Doucet-Jabeuf, et al., "Immunomodulator Activity of Very Low Doses of Thymulin in Mice," *International Journal of Immunotherapy*, 1987, 3: 191–200.

6. V. Daurat, P. Dorfman, and M. Bastide, "Immunomodualtory Activity of Low Doses of Interferon in Mice," *Biomedicine and Pharmacotherapeutics*, 1988, 42: 197–206.

7. Personal Communication. For additional information, see Michael Strange, "AIDS: Some Early Clinical Experience," *British Homoeopathic Journal*, October, 1988, 77: 224–7. Michael Strange, "'AIDS: What Homoeopathy Can Offer," *The Homoeopath: Journal of the Society of Homoeopaths*, 1987, 6,3: 117–124.

8. Bill Gray, "AIDS: A Chronic Multifactorial Miasmataic Disease," *Resonance*, January-February, 1988, 10: 13.

9. Laurence Badgley. Advance Immune Discoveries Symposium. Los Angeles, February 4, 1989. See also L. Badgley, *Journal of the American Institute of Homeopathy*, March, 1987, 80: 8–14.

10. G. F. Lemp, S. Payne, N. Dennese, et al., "Survival Trends for Patients with AIDS," *JAMA*, January 19, 1990, 263, 3: 402–406.

11. Strange, 1988.

12. M. Jenaer, B. Marichal, and A. Doppagne, "Etude cliniqiue preliminaire sur l'efficacité d'un traitement immunotherapique dans le syndrome d'immuno-deficience acquise," *Homeopathie,* June, 1990, 7, 2: 23–28. "Homeopathy and AIDS: Hope or Hype," *Boston Phoenix*, July 21, 1989: 4.

13. Personal Communication.

14. For a general review of research on Hypericum, see Christopher Hobbs, "St. John's Wort (Hypericum perforatum L.)," *HerbalGram*, Fall, 1988, 24–33. See also D. Meruelo, "Therapeutic Agents with Dramatic Antiretroviral Activity and Little Toxicity at Effective Doses: Aromatic Polycyclic Diones Hypericin and Pseudohypericin," *Proceedings of the National Academy of Sciences,* 85: 5230–34.

15. "Hypericum and AIDS," *Medical Herbalism*, January, 1990: 1–2. See also *AIDS Treatment News*, 91, November 17, 1989.

16. L. M. Singh and Girish Gupta, "Antiviral Efficacy of Homoeopathic Drugs Against Animal Viruses," *British Homoeopathic Journal*, 74 (July, 1985): 168–174.

17. R. G. Gibson, et al., "Homoeopathic Therapy in Rheumatoid Arthritis: Evaluation by Double-Blind Clinical Therapeutic Trial," *British Journal of Clinical Pharmacology*, September, 1980: 453–459.

18. See footnote 2.

How to Learn More
About Homeopathy

Virtually anyone can learn about homeopathic principles as well as how to use some of the medicines for common acute, non-life-threatening health problems. After reading this book, you can expand your knowledge by reading other homeopathic books and by attending lectures, workshops, and training programs given in different parts of the United States. You can also learn about homeopathy by obtaining cassette tapes of these programs, by participating in one of the many homeopathic study groups that presently exist, and by joining one or more of the homeopathic organizations.

With a little knowledge of homeopathy, you probably will be pleasantly surprised at how effective you can be in treating some of your own and your family's health problems with homeopathic medicines. There are also limits to what a nonprofessional can treat effectively. There is, for instance, a significant difference in the knowledge about homeopathy needed to treat chronic disease as compared with common nonserious acute conditions.

In order to get the most out of the various homeopathic books, tapes, workshops, study groups, and organizations, you should, first of all, clarify what it is you really want to do with homeopathy. Some people may simply want to know a little about homeopathy's principles and then go to a professional homeopath for treatment. Others may want to learn to treat themselves for simple acute conditions. Others will want to study more deeply and master the nuances of the homeopathic constitutional types. And still others will want to learn about the history of homeopathy, its research, its cosmology, and its similarities to and differences

236

from other therapies. Once you are clear about the direction you are interested in taking, it is more likely that you will get there.

Starting Off

Before learning how to use the homeopathic medicines, it is important to first understand homeopathic philosophy. This book has introduced many of the key principles, but more extensive knowledge can be obtained by reading George Vithoulkas's *Homeopathy: Medicine of the New Man;* the more sophisticated reader can get his *Science of Homeopathy.*

Other basic books on homeopathic philosophy are Dr. Samuel Hahnemann's *Organon of Medicine* and Dr. James Tyler Kent's *Lectures on Homoeopathic Philosophy.* Hahnemann's book was the seminal work on homeopathy, and it is not only of historical importance but of particular value today in understanding homeopathic philosophy.* Kent later summarized Hahnemann's *Organon* and added some of his own interpretations to homeopathy. Although his *Lectures* were written in 1900, they are still ahead of their time.

The three best homeopathic self-care books are Stephen Cummings and Dana Ullman's *Everybody's Guide to Homeopathic Medicines,* Dr. Maesimund Panos and Jane Heimlich's *Homeopathic Medicine at Home,* and Dr. David Gemmell's *Everyday Homeopathy.* The Cummings-Ullman book provides more depth and breadth on how to individualize the homeopathic medicines, while the Panos-Heimlich book describes much of the authors' experiences with homeopathy and is written in a somewhat chatty fashion, making for easy reading. The Gemmell book discusses the homeopathic treatment of more conditions than the other two books, though it does not provide much individualizing detail about each medicine. It is basically recommended that the reader use these and other books together to get the most information for home care.

Other self-care guides that should be considered are Dr.

---

*The last edition of *The Organon*, its sixth, was written just before Hahnemann's death in 1843, but was not published until 1921.

Alonzo Shadman's *Who Is Your Doctor and Why,* Dr. Trevor Smith's *Homoeopathic Medicines: A Doctor's Guide to Remedies for Common Ailments,* Dr. Trevor Smith's *A Woman's Guide to Homeopathic Medicines,* D. M. Gibson's *Homoeopathy in Accidents and Injuries,* and Dr. Dorothy Shepherd's *Homoeopathy for the First Aider.*

To refine your prescribing, it is helpful to obtain Dr. William Boericke's *Pocket Manual of Materia Medica with Repertory.* A "materia medica" provides detailed information on the various symptoms that a substance has been found to cause in overdose and thus to cure in microdose. Boericke's materia medica presents the symptoms of each medicine in outline fashion for easy and quick use. A "repertory" is a listing of symptoms and those substances that have been found to cause and cure each symptom. For instance, one would use a repertory to look for a compilation of those medicines that are good for headaches that occur in the front of the head in the morning (in the "head" section, under the subsection "pain," under the further subsection "frontal pain worse in the morning"). After reviewing a sick person's various symptoms in the repertory, one can then obtain more detailed information about each of the possible medicines by looking them up in a materia medica. A repertory and a materia medica complement each other. Boericke's book serves as a good materia medica and repertory for the beginner.

There is now a fair amount of easily accessible homeopathic material on cassette tapes. Homeopathic Educational Services (2124 Kittredge St., Berkeley, CA 94704) sells a comprehensive assortment of tapes on homeopathic philosophy and self-care. Better than simply listening to lectures is attending courses, such as those offered by the National Center for Homeopathy (1500 Massachusetts Ave., N.W., Washington, D.C. 20005). This organization offers annual courses to the general public on how to learn to use homeopathic medicines at home.

The interested reader may join homeopathic organizations in order to keep informed of the latest information in the field and to learn about current educational opportunities. (See "Homeopathic Organizations" later in Part III for a list of these organizations.)

It is also possible to participate in a homeopathic study group, if there is one nearby. Contact the National Center for Homeopathy for a list of study groups in the United States. (Also, see "Starting and Participating in a Homeopathic Study Group" later in this section.)

The Next Step

After becoming familiar with the introductory information about homeopathy, a student has many options from which to learn more. He or she can choose to explore homeopathic methodology (case-taking and case analysis); homeopathic history, research, and cosmology; or the subtleties of the homeopathic medicines themselves.

Homeopathic Methodology: Books on homeopathic methodology are similar to those on homeopathic philosophy, though the former describe in greater detail how to practice homeopathy. Excellent books on this subject include Dr. Herbert Roberts's *The Principles and Art of Cure by Homoeopathy*, Dr. M. L. Dhawale's *The Principles and Practice of Homoeopathy* (a 600-page book that provides the most detailed information presently available on the subject), Dr. Elizabeth Hubbard Wright's *A Brief Study Course in Homoeopathy* (a superb, short overview), and Dr. Richard Crews's *Introductory Workbook in Homeopathy* (a suitable workbook that is good for individuals and study groups). The newest significant title, which will probably become a leading textbook, is Dr. Gerhard Koehler's *The Handbook of Homoeopathy*.

Homeopathic History: Homeopathic principles of healing predate Hippocrates and have been utilized in many cultures throughout the world. In three monumental volumes on Western medical history, collectively entitled *Divided Legacy*, Dr. Harris Coulter documents the birth and development of homeopathic and "empirical" principles and their historical conflict with conventional "rational" medical practice. Volume 1 concentrates on medical history from Hippocrates to Paracelsus (350 B.C through the 1500s). Volume 2 focuses on European medicine from the 1600s to the 1850s (and, in so doing, covers the initial and early developments of homeopathy). Volume 3 details American medical history from 1800 to 1914 and chronicles the serious conflict that homeopathy experienced with the American Medical Association.

Richard Grossinger's *Planet Medicine: From Stone-Age Shamanism to Post-Industrial Healing* is only one-fourth about homeopathy, but Grossinger, an anthropologist, describes homeopathy in the light of historical, evolutionary, and scientific developments. He shows how homeopathy represents a bridge between the ancient healing methods and modern scientific healing practices, and he raises many of the questions that newcomers to the topic first ask. This book is useful to readers trying to place homeopathy in a wider cultural and philosophical framework.

People interested in an excellent account of the life and times of Samuel Hahnemann can read Dr. Trevor Cook's *Samuel Hahnemann*. Anthony Campbell's *Two Faces of Homoeopathy* describes the two major ways in which homeopathy has developed both in thought and practice: mystical and scientific. Although Campbell clearly has his own biases about what he calls scientific, his book raises some important questions for serious students and practitioners of homeopathy.

Homeopathic Research: Most people are not aware of the legacy of competent research in homeopathy. Dr. Harris Coulter's *Homoeopathic Science and Modern Medicine* reviews the field in the context of research and modern scientific understanding. Dana Ullman's *Monograph of Homeopathic Research* (volumes 1 and 2) compiles laboratory and clinical studies that have been published in conventional medical and scientific journals as well as in homeopathic publications. Articles on theoretical extrapolations about how the medicines might work are also included.

Drawing from the cutting edge of physics and chemistry, Drs. Gerhard Resch and Viktor Gutmann have written *The Scientific Foundations of Homeopathy*, a highly technical analysis of how the homeopathic microdoses have biological action and clinical efficacy. Dr. Resch is a physician and homeopath, while Dr. Gutmann is a professor of chemistry, and together they have published numerous articles in respected scientific journals.

Homeopathic Cosmology: Only one book fits completely under this heading. Dr. Edward C. Whitmont's *Psyche and Substance: Essays on Homeopathy in the Light of Jungian Psychology* is unique in the way in which it blends the basic premises of homeopathy with Jungian psychology, alchemy, and new physics. Besides discussing the relationships and the connections between mind, body, and nature, Dr. Whitmont describes a dozen common homeopathic medicines and the "bodymind archetypal personality" that each of these medicines is known to treat. This book may be difficult for the uninitiated, but its insights are profound and its implications significant.

Matthew Wood's *Seven Herbs: Plants as Teachers* is in part a materia medica of seven herbs (only two of which are commonly used homeopathic medicines) and in part a cosmological description of how herbs play a special role in healing human ailments and in teaching us about ourselves. The author synthesizes the wisdom of Paracelsus, the science of homeopathy, and the stories of the Bible to help us understand how to apply these herbs.

Homeopathic Medicines: After learning the basics of homeopathy, some people love to study various homeopathic medicines as a way of finding their own and their friends' constitutional medicine. Although it is not recommended that one self-prescribe a constitutional medicine, it is still a useful mental exercise. The process of reading about the various typologies and of finding the appropriate one is a mixture of detective work, self-discovery, rational analysis, and intuitive assessment.

Catherine Coulter's *Portraits of Homoeopathic Medicines* discusses nine of the key constitutional types, eloquently describing them in terms of well-known characters from the classics in literature, from famous personalities, and from Jungian archetypes.*

Other materia medicas are less poetic than *Portraits* but also provide valuable details and insights necessary for accurate prescribing. Some of the better materia medicas are: Dr. James Tyler Kent's *Lectures on Homoeopathic Materia Medica*, Dr. Margaret Tyler's *Drug Pictures*, Dr. D. M. Gibson's *Studies of Homoeopathic Remedies*, Dr. Charles Wheeler's *An Introduction to the Principles and Practice of Homoeopathy*, and Dr. John Clarke's

---

*There are, of course, many more than nine constitutional types, and Ms. Coulter is presently compiling further volumes of her work.

Dictionary of Practical Materia Medica.

Complementing the materia medicas are repertories. The single best repertory is still Dr. James Tyler Kent's *Repertory of Homoeopathic Materia Medica.* This is an invaluable text for any serious student or practitioner of homeopathy.

Books on clinical homeopathy describe common health problems and the homeopathic medicines most regularly found to be effective in treating them. Although these books seem to make homeopathy easier to practice, they often do not provide enough individualizing information necessary to prescribe the correct medicine. Still, there are some excellent books of clinical homeopathy, including Dr. Margery Blackie's new *Classical Homoeopathy,* Dr. Prakash Vakil's *Diseases of the Cardiovascular System: A Textbook of Homoeopathic Therapeutics* and his *Central Nervous System: A Textbook of Homoeopathic Therapeutics.* Other useful texts are Dr. D. M. Borland's *Homoeopathy in Practice,* Dr. Colin Lessell's *Homoeopathy for Physicians,* Dr. Trevor Smith's *The Homoeopathic Treatment of Emotional Illnesses,* Dr. Richard Hughes's *Principles and Practice of Homoeopathy,* Dr. Colin Lessell's *The Dental Prescriber,* and Dr. Jacques Jouanny's *Essentials of Homoeopathic Therapeutics.*

Homeopaths believe in small doses of medicines, but not small doses of books. Homeopathic books provide the collected experiences of two centuries by physicians and laypersons. Since homeopathy is both a science and an art, these books combine the intricate clinical detail of the homeopathic medicines with special insights about the healing process.

Starting and Participating in a Homeopathic Study Group

Ever since the origins of homeopathic medicine, informal study groups have been one of the traditional methods of transmitting information on homeopathy. Even at homeopathic medical schools in the 1800s, students and faculty members met outside of the classroom to study homeopathy together. Occasionally, laypersons also participated in these study groups, but more often they organized their own groups.

Such professional and lay groups are still quite common today. They provide a forum for people to share their thoughts and questions about homeopathic philosophy and methodology, their understanding of how and when to prescribe the medicines, and their experience with homeopathy. Groups tend to be helpful in guiding people to the best books and articles, and through the complicated process of studying homeopathic materia medicas, repertories, and the art of case-taking. Of particular importance, the study sessions provide a support group for people who are involved in this distinctly different type of medical practice. This kind of support group is sometimes very important to members, since their doctors, colleagues, and friends can be very critical of homeopathy, whether these people have knowledge of it or not.

If there is no homeopathic study group in your area, or if there is a group but you want to create another one, there are several tried and true ways you can get started. One effective way to start a study group is to invite a nearby homeopath to give a public lecture on homeopathy. Publicize the lecture through flyers and press releases.

Since a large number of people interested in homeopathy have children and are looking for alternatives to conventional medicine, it is a good idea to post flyers for a lecture or for your study group at local child-care facilities, public schools, PTA meetings, YMCAs, public swimming pools, churches, temples, community organization offices, and numerous other places where children and their parents go.

As for press coverage, you will be surprised at how easy it is to get your activity listed in numerous local newspapers. You may also be able to get one of the local papers to write an article that can both promote homeopathy and advertise the lecture.*

Inform those in attendance at the lecture that a study group is being formed and that they are welcome to participate. Hopefully, the lecture will inspire them enough to want to learn more. Make certain to obtain the names, addresses, and phone numbers of all those who attend the lecture so that they can be kept informed about upcoming study group meetings and future homeopathic lectures.

Besides giving occasional public lectures, some homeopaths attend study group meetings. Since most study group meetings will probably not have a homeopath in attendance, one or two members of the group should keep a list of questions or concerns that the group has raised in previous meetings so that these can be discussed with the homeopath.

There are numerous excellent cassette tapes on various subjects in homeopathy that are very helpful to study groups. Groups of people can listen to a tape together. The facilitator of the meeting can occasionally stop the tape to encourage discussion on certain important points. Some parts of the tape can be listened to more than once, since the lecturer may be making complex but important points. Cassette tapes can also be very helpful to groups that are unable to get a local homeopath to lecture. For a list of lectures on tape, contact Homeopathic Educational Services (2124

---

*To learn more about how to write press releases, public service announcements, and other means of getting media exposure, I highly recommend the *Media How-To Notebook*. For a copy of this valuable workbook, send $6.00 to: Media Alliance, Fort Mason, Building D, Laguna and Marina Sts., San Francisco, CA 94123.

Kittredge St., Berkeley, CA 94704).

It is also a good idea to have introductory articles on homeopathy and brochures about how to obtain homeopathic books and tapes at all public lectures and at study group meetings. Brochures from the various homeopathic organizations provide good information about homeopathy. Request a stack of brochures from sources of homeopathic books, tapes, and medicines. Homeopathic Educational Services has useful introductory articles on homeopathy that may, with permission, be duplicated for distribution.

Between guest appearances by local homeopaths and/or cassette tape lectures, study groups can choose to discuss a particular chapter or a couple of chapters from a homeopathic book. It is best to decide in advance which chapter everyone should read. It is also very helpful to choose a facilitator for the meeting. The facilitator will study the chapter(s) with particular care so that he or she will be able to ask essential questions to elicit the deepest understanding of the material. The group will generally be more successful if the facilitator actively seeks the group's participation in discussion. It is also worthwhile to take turns being the facilitator.

Once your group gets going, you might consider studying the homeopathic materia medicas. Most homeopaths recommend that only one medicine be studied at a time. The chosen medicine should be studied as thoroughly as possible. You should each read about it in several materia medicas, and you might consider reading the material numerous times.

Since materia medicas are full of detailed information about a medicine, it is necessary to study each medicine in a systematic way so that you can retain as much information about it as possible. Each person develops his or her own systematic way of studying a materia medica. One common method is to summarize the general symptoms and the particular symptoms on an index card or a sheet of paper.* In general, students of homeopathy learn the medicine most effectively when they try to memorize key features of the medicine and when they get a deep feeling about it.

---

*"General symptoms" are experienced by the entire body (e.g., feeling cold or restless), whereas "particular symptoms" are experienced in a particular part of the body (e.g., having cold or restless feet).

Some people make up mnemonic devices. Others may meditate on a medicine's characteristics. Some people even make drawings of the person who would typically need this medicine. And some people dramatize the medicine in a short play. It is good to encourage study group members to discuss a medicine without the use of their notes, and ultimately to check with notes only when someone questions the accuracy of a symptom or at the end of the discussion.

One systematic way to learn about a medicine in a study group is to discuss its most characteristic symptoms first. Afterwards, there should be discussion of the psychological symptoms, then noteworthy general physical symptoms, then noteworthy particular physical symptoms, and finally the less characteristic physical symptoms. When discussing the physical symptoms, it is helpful to talk about them in the order of head to toe.

Studying the homeopathic repertories in a group can be fun. It is common for new students and even experienced homeopaths to have difficulty finding certain symptoms anywhere in the repertory. Getting a group of people to find a symptom can be a game, the winner being the first person to find it. It is also interesting for a person to give the group a list of symptoms as an exercise to see how many people find all of them. These games can be a playful and effective way to learn.

Another way to learn about homeopathy is to practice homeopathic case-taking. Study groups can consider having one person take another person's case in front of the group and then give the interviewer feedback about his or her ability to elicit symptoms. People who agree to have their case taken should know beforehand that they will be asked intimate questions about their health and life. Participants in such discussions must agree to full confidentiality, and nothing about the person's case should be discussed with others.

Study groups can also consider breaking down into pairs of people who exchange turns taking each other's case. People quickly realize how much they don't know when they first try case-taking. This experience is extremely valuable in learning the nuances of interviewing a person to determine his or her homeopathic medicine.

Depending upon the study group's collective degree of knowledge, there are some cases that may be too complex for its members. Generally, people with acute, non-life-threatening illnesses are perfect for study group discussion, whereas people with chronic diseases should be seen by a medical professional. Stephen Cummings and Dana Ullman's *Everybody's Guide to Homeopathic Medicines* and certain medical reference books provide some guidelines for when medical care is recommended and when various home-care measures can be considered safe.

Discussing cases from outside the study group can also be very instructive, for there is a tendency in study groups to talk only about one's own cured cases. Although discussion of successes will help the group's members to learn a medicine's effectiveness, discussion of medicines that did not work is also instructive in learning how to prescribe. Even discussion of prescriptions that have uncertain effectiveness can provide helpful lessons in learning about homeopathic care.

As you probably have determined from this discussion of study groups, there is much value in studying homeopathy with others. Besides providing a fine opportunity to learn about homeopathy, these groups also introduce you to a great group of people with whom friendships develop that provide their own special healing.

Beyond Books and Study Groups

In addition to learning homeopathy through books and study groups, it is recommended that all those seriously interested in learning about homeopathy attend the various homeopathic conferences and training programs and join all or most of the homeopathic organizations in order to be kept up-to-date on the various educational opportunities. The following list of homeopathic organizations, pharmacies, and schools and training programs will be of special value to you.

There are also various less well known newsletters and publications on homeopathy. Contact Homeopathic Educational Services for this list. Homeopathic Educational Services also has some information about training programs outside the United States.

Whether one chooses to dive deeply into homeopathy or to

swim slowly into it, the benefits of this art and science will sink in one way or another and change your understanding of healing. Once smitten by knowledge of homeopathy, you will find it hard to settle for anything else.

The National Center for Homeopathy coordinates the activities of over 100 study groups in the United States. To discover if there is a homeopathic study group in your area and for more information on how to start one yourself, contact:

National Center for Homeopathy
801 N. Fairfax #306
Alexandria, VA 22314

Sources of Books, Tapes, and General Information on Homeopathy

HOMEOPATHIC EDUCATIONAL SERVICES, 2124 Kittredge St., Berkeley, CA 94704

Homeopathic Educational Services is the most comprehensive source of homeopathic books, tapes, medicines, software, and general information.

Homeopathic Manufacturers

Many of the homeopathic manufacturers also sell homeopathic books.

BIOLOGICAL HOMEOPATHIC INDUSTRIES, 11600 Cochiti S.E., Albuquerque, NM 87123.

BOERICKE AND TAFEL, 2381 Circadian Way, Santa Rosa, CA 95407.

BOIRON-BORNEMANN, INC., 1208 Amosland Road, Norwood, PA 19074; also: 98c W. Cochran, Simi Valley, CA 93065.

DOLISOS, 3014 Rigel, Las Vegas, NV 89102.

LONGEVITY PURE MEDICINES, 9595 Wilshire Blvd. #706, Beverly Hills, CA 90212.

LUYTIES PHARMACAL, 4200 Laclede Ave., St. Louis, MO 63108.

STANDARD HOMEOPATHIC COMPANY, 204–210 W. 131st St., Los Angeles, CA 90061.

Homeopathic Organizations

NATIONAL CENTER FOR HOMEOPATHY, 801 N. Fairfax #306, Alexandria, VA 22314.

AMERICAN INSTITUTE OF HOMEOPATHY, 1585 Glencoe St. #44, Denver CO 80220.

INTERNATIONAL FOUNDATION FOR HOMEOPATHY, 2366 Eastlake Ave. E. #301, Seattle, WA 98102.

FOUNDATION FOR HOMEOPATHIC EDUCATION AND RESEARCH, 5916 Chabot Crest, Oakland, CA 94618.

AMERICAN ASSOCIATION OF HOMEOPATHIC PHARMACISTS, P.O. Box 2273, Falls Church, VA 22042.

BOIRON RESEARCH INSTITUTE, 1208 Amosland Road, Norwood, PA 19074.

BRITISH HOMOEOPATHIC ASSOCIATION, The Royal London Homoeopathic Hospital, Great Ormond St., London WC1N 3HR, England.

THE SOCIETY OF HOMOEOPATHS, 2 Artizan Road, Northampton NN1 4HU, England.

*Schools and Training Programs in North America**

NATIONAL CENTER FOR HOMEOPATHY, 801 N. Fairfax #306, Alexandria, VA 22314.

INTERNATIONAL FOUNDATION FOR HOMEOPATHY, 2366 Eastlake Ave. E. #301, Seattle, WA 98102.

HAHNEMANN COLLEGE OF HOMEOPATHY, 1918 Milvia St., Berkeley, CA 94704.

JOHN BASTYR COLLEGE OF NATUROPATHIC MEDICINE, 1408 N.E. 45th St., Seattle, WA 98105.

NATIONAL COLLEGE OF NATUROPATHIC MEDICINE, 11231 S.E. Market St., Portland, OR 97216.

ONTARIO COLLEGE OF NATUROPATHIC MEDICINE, 60 Berl Avenue, Toronto, Ontario, Canada.

PACIFIC ACADEMY OF HOMEOPATHIC MEDICINE, 1678 Shattuck #42, Berkeley, CA 94709.

---

*For updated listings of addresses and phone numbers of schools and training programs, contact Homeopathic Educational Services, 2124 Kittredge St., Berkeley, CA 94704.

INTERNATIONAL COLLEGE OF HOMEOPATHIC AND BIO-
DYNAMIC STUDIES, 11423–25 Crenshaw Blvd., Inglewood,
CA 90303.
NEW ENGLAND SCHOOL OF HOMEOPATHY, 356 Middle St.,
Amherst, MA 01002.
HAHNEMANN ACADEMY OF NORTH AMERICA, 2801 Rodeo
Road #B-135, Santa Fe, NM 87505.
NATIONAL HOMEOPATHIC DENTAL SEMINARS, P.O. Box
123, Marengo, IL 60152.
HOMEOPATHIC VETERINARY COURSES, c/o Richard Pitcairn,
DVM, Ph.D., 1283 Lincoln St., Eugene, OR 97404.

Introductory and Self-Care Books

Cummings, Stephen, and Dana Ullman. *Everybody's Guide to Homeo-
pathic Medicines.* Los Angeles: Jeremy Tarcher, 1984/1991.
Hammond, Christopher. *How to Use Homeopathy Effectively.* Not-
tingham, England: Caritas, 1988.
Kruzel, Thomas. *The Acute Homeopathic Prescriber.* Berkeley: North
Atlantic, (forthcoming in 1992).
Neustaedter, Randall. *The Immunization Decision: A Guide for Par-
ents.* Berkeley: North Atlantic, 1990.
Panos, Maesimund, and Jane Heimlich. *Homeopathic Medicine at
Home.* Los Angeles: J.P. Tarcher, 1980.
Richardson, Sarah. *Homeopathy: An Illustrated Guide.* New York:
Harmony, 1988.
Schmidt, Michael A. *Childhood Ear Infections: What Every Parent
and Physician Should Know about Their Prevention, Home Care,
and Alternative Treatments.* Berkeley: North Atlantic, 1990.
Smith, Trevor. *Homeopathic Medicines for Women.* Rochester, Vt.:
Healing Arts, 1989.
Subotnick, Steven. *Sports and Exercise Injuries: Conventional,
Homeopathic, and Alternative Treatments.* Berkeley: North At-
lantic, 1991.
Ullman, Dana. *The Homeopathic Treatment of Our Infants and Chil-
dren.* Los Angeles: Jeremy Tarcher (to be published in 1992).
Vithoulkas, George. *Homeopathy: Medicine for the New Man.* New
York: Arco, 1979.

Philosophy, Methodology, and Research

Coulter, Harris L. *Homoeopathic Science and Modern Medicine: The Physics of Healing with Microdoses*. Berkeley: North Atlantic, 1981.

Dhawale, M. L. *Principles and Practice of Homoeopathy*. Bombay: D. K. Homoeopathic Corporation, 1967.

Hahnemann, Samuel. *Organon of Medicine*. Los Angeles, J. P. Tarcher, 1982. Reprint.

Kent, James Tyler. *Lectures on Homoeopathic Philosophy*. Berkeley: North Atlantic, 1979. Reprint.

Koehler, Gerhard. *The Handbook of Homeopathy*. Rochester, Vt.: Healing Arts, 1987.

Roberts, H. A. *The Principles and Art of Cure by Homoeopathy*. New Delhi: B. Jain. Reprint.

Vithoulkas, George. *The Science of Homeopathy*. New York: Grove, 1979.

Wright, Elizabeth Hubbard. *A Brief Study Course in Homeopathy*. St. Louis: Formur, 1977.

Materia Medicas and Repertories

Allen, H. C. *Keynotes and Characteristic of the Materica Medica*. New Delhi: B. Jain. Reprint.

Boericke, William. *Pocket Manual of Materia Medica with Repertory*. Santa Rosa: Boericke and Tafel. Reprint.

Clarke, John. *Dictionary of Practical Materia Medica* (3 volumes). Essex, England: C. W. Daniel. Reprint.

Coulter, Catherine. *Portraits of Homoeopathic Medicines* (2 volumes). Berkeley: North Atlantic, 1986, 1988.

Gibson, D. M. *Studies of Homoeopathic Remedies*. Beaconsfield, England: Beaconsfield Publishers, 1987.

Herscu, Paul. *The Homeopathic Treatment of Children: Pediatric Constitutional Types*. Berkekley: North Atlantic, 1991.

Kent, James Tyler. *Lectures on Homoeopathic Materia Medica*. New Delhi: B. Jain. Reprint.

Kent, James Tyler. *Repertory of Homoeopathic Materia Medica*. New Delhi: B. Jain. Reprint.

Nash, E. B. *Leaders in Homoeopathic Therapeutics*. New Delhi: B. Jain. Reprint.

Tyler, Margaret. *Drug Pictures*. Essex, England: C. W. Daniel, 1952.

Wheeler, Charles. *An Introduction to the Principles and Practice of Homoeopathy*. New Delhi: B Jain. Reprint.

Whitmont, Edward C. *Psyche and Substance: Essays on Homeopathy in the Light of Jungian Psychology*. Berkeley: North Atlantic, 1980.

History of Homeopathy

Coulter, Harris L. *Divided Legacy: A History of the Schism in Medical Thought* (3 volumes). Berkeley: North Atlantic, 1975, 1977, 1981. Of special interest is volume III: *Divided Legacy: The Conflict Between Homoeopathy and the American Medical Association*.

Grossinger, Richard. *Planet Medicine: From Stone-Age Shamanism to Post-Industrial Medicine*. Berkeley: North Atlantic, 1987.

Handley, Rima. *A Homeopathic Love Story*. Berkeley: North Atlantic, 1990.

Nichols, Philip. *Homoeopathy and the Medical Profession*. Beckenham, England: Croom Helm, 1988.

Finding a Homeopathic Practitioner

Most homeopaths in the United States are medical doctors who have added homeopathic training to their medical studies. There are also a growing number of other health professionals (physician assistants, nurses, dentists, podiatrists, naturopaths, chiropractors, psychologists, and numerous others) who have begun to practice homeopathy. It is generally legal for these practitioners to prescribe homeopathic medicines in the states in which they are licensed, though there are some restrictions. Physician assistants and nurses are allowed only to recommend homeopathic medicines when doing so under the supervision of a physician. Dentists and podiatrists can utilize homeopathic medicines for the respective care and treatment of dental or podiatric conditions. Chiropractors can utilize homeopathic medicines in certain states if they prescribe them as part of the care and treatment of a person's spine. It is uncertain if psychologists are legally permitted to prescribe homeopathic medicines, but it has been conjectured that they can if they do so with the primary intent of treating the person's psychological state rather than physical pathology.

Some laypersons have begun to study and practice homeopathy, and some of these people are excellent practitioners. The legal issues surrounding their practice are not yet clearly defined.

Homeopathic Educational Services and the National Center for Homeopathy sell a directory of licensed health professionals in the United States who practice homeopathy. However, since this list is incomplete, you should talk to people in your own area (friends, health food store owners, community organizations, and so on).

In England there are medical doctors who have become homeopaths (contact the Faculty of Homoeopathy directory; its address is included under "Homeopathic Organizations," above), and there are a new breed of "professional homeopaths" who are not medically trained but who have attended a three-year program of homeopathic training (contact the Society of Homoeopaths for a directory).

There is no foolproof way to find out if a practitioner is good, but here are some helpful guidelines:

1. Find out how much time the practitioner spends with patients. The first visit should be at least one hour, and follow-ups should generally be about twenty or thirty minutes. Less than that may mean that the practitioner does not spend enough time individualizing the correct medicine for you.

2. Find out if the practitioner uses one or more than one medicine at a time. Although there are different ways to practice homeopathy, most experienced practitioners prescribe only one medicine at a time. Good homeopaths prescribe one medicine for the totality of the person's symptoms and do not usually prescribe one medicine for one disease, a second for another, and so on. There are, however, exceptions to this rule. If you hear that numerous people have received good treatment from a practitioner who uses many medicines, this practitioner may be particularly good with this less traditional approach to homeopathy.

3. Does the practitioner ask you about the totality of your physical, emotional, and mental symptoms? If the practitioner does not ask about your psychological state in reasonable detail, or if he or she focuses entirely on your psychological state, seek a practitioner who is interested in the totality of who you are.

It may be necessary to travel some distance to find a good homeopath. This trip may, however, save you many trips to a hospital.

A Note of Prediction
and Caution

It is inevitable that interest in homeopathic medicine will grow in significant ways during the coming years. Its growth will probably outstrip the number of health professionals who presently practice homeopathy or who can get adequate training to use the medicines in a competent way.*

Homeopathy is not a system of health care that a health professional can learn simply by taking a weekend workshop, or even several weekend workshops. One should expect to study homeopathy over a couple of years to begin to master it, and even then its study is lifelong. Learning the depth and breadth of homeopathy is greatly aided by having a good teacher. (See "Schools and Training Programs in the United States," above, for accessing such training.)

Although it takes much time and dedication to learn to use the medicines to treat chronic conditions, one can fairly quickly learn to use the medicines for acute conditions. There are several good books that can teach virtually anyone to use the homeopathic medicines at home for simple, self-limiting acute conditions. These books teach people how to use a homeopathic medicine kit at home.

Beginners are often impressed by their successes in using the homeopathic medicines. Even better results are obtained by those who study the system in depth and who develop increasing experiences with the medicines.

---

*Most homeopaths already have very busy practices, and some have become so busy that they only accept new patients on rare occasions.

It seems probable that the rapid growth of homeopathy may lead some health professionals to practice homeopathy before they are very competent at it. Patients who then experience this type of homeopathy may not be very impressed by the results they experience. Such care will not be a measure of the ineffectiveness of homeopathy, but of the limited knowledge and experience of the practitioner.

Inevitably there will be some confusion in the public mind as to who is a "qualified" practitioner of homeopathy. This same confusion occurs in the development and popularization of any professional specialty. Hopefully, those citizens who feel that homeopathy offers a special service in healing the ills of humankind will help the various homeopathic and consumer organizations to educate the public on how, when, and where quality homeopathic care can be obtained.

A good way to ensure that one is receiving quality homeopathic care is to become educated in the system oneself. Informed consumers can do much to aid in their own treatment.

Homeopathy's founder Samuel Hahnemann frequently challenged his critics by saying, "Aude sapere," which, translated from Latin, means "dare to taste, to understand, to experience." Hahnemann and other homeopaths since his time have asserted that it is not enough to criticize homeopathy on the ground that it does not *seem* that it should work. The proof of homeopathy is in its practice. One must try it oneself. Whatever efforts it takes to learn to use the medicines in acute care or to find a good practitioner to treat one's chronic condition, such efforts are a "healthy investment."

Index

Abdomen (also see Stomach), 86, 103, 114, 117, 167–169, 207
Abdominal gas, 78, 102, 206
Abrams, Dr. Albert, 24
Abscesses, 56, 211, 212
Accidents, 100
Aches (see Pain)
Achilles tendonitis, 178
Acids, 97, 98, 114
Acne (also see Skin), 108
Aconite (monkshood), 81, 87, 94, 95, 129, 130, 211
Actaea racemosa (cimicifuga or black snakeroot), 61, 84, 110
Acupressure, 175
Acupuncture/Acupuncturists, xx, 18, 23, 48, 50, 175, 210, 220, 247
Acute conditions (also see Chronic conditions), xvi, xviii, xx, 20, 22, 27, 43, 49, 51, 71, 79, 80, 83, 88, 100, 109, 110, 112, 121, 127, 128, 129, 144, 145, 146, 154, 210, 250, 251
Acute medicines (also see Constitutional medicines; Fundamental medicines), 19, 80, 81, 127, 144
Adaptive responses, 5
Addiction, 186, 187, 194, 196
Adelaide, Queen, 29
Adrenal gland, 114, 115
Africa, 132, 134
AIDS (Acquired Immune Deficiency Syndrome), xiv, 128, 132, 133, 134, 135
Aikido, 8
Albright, Dr. S.A.., 206
Alchemy, 7, 233
Alcohol/Alcoholism, 12, 15, 81, 93, 117, 162, 186, 194, 196, 202
Alcott, Louisa May, 40
Allergens, 6, 64, 140, 142
Allergies (also see Asthma; Exzema; Hay Fever; Overreactions), xv, xx, 6, 14, 64, 98, 139–151, 188
Allergy shots (see Injections)
Allium cepa (onion), 130, 144
Allopathy/Allopathists (also see Conventional medicine), 40, 42, 126, 219

"Alternative medicine" (also see Complementary medicine; Conventional medicine; Natural therapies), xviii, xxiii, 18, 48, 49, 220
Alumina (aluminum), 131
Aluminum, 162–163, 207
Alzheimer's disease, 163, 207
American Academy of Allergy, 143
American Cancer Society, 219
American Academy of Pediatrics, 75, 92, 93
American College of Obstetrics and Gynecology (ACOG), 73
American Council for Life Insurance, 219
American Dental Association (ADA), 205, 206, 207, 209
American Institute of Homeopathy, 37, 41, 185, 243
American Medical Association (AMA), 36, 37, 38, 39, 41, 44, 47, 107, 232
Amalgam fillings, 208–211
American Psychiatric Association, 186
American Society of Dental Surgeons (ASDS), 208
Ammonia, 74
Ammonium muriaticum (ammonium chloride), 179
Amniotomy, 75, 76
Amphetamines, 6, 101, 107
Amyl nitrate, 132
Anacardium (marking nut), 178
Analgesia/Analgesics, 61, 76, 83
Anemia, 25, 78, 79, 204
Anesthesia, 76, 77, 83, 96
Anger (also see Emotions), 16, 21, 22, 110, 190, 194
Animals, xvii, 56, 62, 63, 66, 84, 139, 142, 149
Ankles (also see Legs), 178, 181
Anorexia, 115, 194
Antacid pills, 163
Antibiotics, xv, xviii, xix, 25, 87, 91, 92, 95, 111, 119, 120, 121, 122, 123, 124, 125, 126, 127, 129, 132, 133, 134, 135, 136
Antibodies, 6, 87, 93, 140
Antidepressants (also see Depression; Tranquilizers), 107, 188
Antidotes, 28
Antihistamines (also see *Histamine*), 59, 93, 140, 141, 159

Antimonium crudum (black sulphide of antimony), 100
Antimonium tart (tartar emetic), 86, 100
Antipsychotic medications, 188
Antiviral agents (also see Viruses), 5, 64, 128, 130, 135
Anus, 133
Anxiety (see Fear)
Apis mellifica (crushed bee), 8, 63, 64, 111, 118, 127, 145, 178, 179
Apothecaries (see Pharmacists)
Appetite (see Eating)
Applied kinesiology, 24
Arbor vitae (see *Thuja*)
ARC (AIDS-related complex), 134, 135
Argenticum nitricum (silver nitrate), 101, 102
Argentina, 18, 29
Arms, 76, 86, 88
Arnica (mountain daisy), 60, 61, 84, 85, 86, 100, 177, 178, 179
Arsenicum album (arsenic), 19, 21, 36, 62, 98, 100, 101, 102, 127, 131, 134, 192–194
Arteries (also see Blood; Capillaries; Veins), 156
Arthritis, 6, 10, 17, 26, 59, 61, 135, 164
Asphyxiation (also see Breathing), 86
Aspirin, 5, 64, 93, 94, 154, 175, 214, 222
Asthma (also see Allergies), 17, 25, 99, 139, 142, 143, 146, 147, 150, 176, 191
Atoms (also see Ions; Molecules; Protons; Subatomic activity), 13
Atropine, 142
"Attention deficit disorders" (see Hyperactivity)
Attention span, 102
Australia, 50
Austria, 40
Autoimmune diseases, 164
Avena sativa (oat), 131
Aversions (also see Allergies), 19, 148
Avogadro's Law, 13

Babies (see Children)
Back problems, 9, 79, 114, 180
Bacteria (also see Disease; Germs; Viruses), xv, xviii, xix, 4, 5, 64, 86, 119, 120, 121, 122, 127, 128, 129, 131, 132, 135, 203, 204, 205, 215
Badiaga (freshwater sponge), 135
Baking soda, 97
Balance/Imbalance, 108, 110, 122, 144
Baldwin, Dr. George, 213
Barberry (see *Berberis*)
Barbiturates, 142
Barnes, Joseph K., 38
Barr, Sir James, 24
Basophils, 64
Baum, Michael, xxiv
B-cells (also see Immune system; T-cells), 134
Bees, crushed (see *Apis mellifica*)
Bee stings/venom, 142, 145
Behavioral tendencies/problems, 18, 19, 21, 93, 94, 97, 103, 189
Behring, Dr. Emil Adolph von, 6
Belgium/Belgians, 50, 82
Belladonna (deadly nightshade), 59, 84, 87, 88, 94, 95, 100, 110, 127, 129, 130, 142, 212, 214
Bellis perrenis (daisy), 86, 178
Berberis (barberry), 111
Bernard, Claude, 122
Bible, 234
Bezold, Clement, xvi
Bichromate of potash (see *Kali bichromicum*)
Biochemistry (also see Chemistry), 63
Bioenergetic force/process, 15, 65
Biofeedback, 219
Biological effects, 55, 56, 57, 58, 63, 65
Biology/Biologists (also see Microbiology), 13, 119
"Bioplasm," 15
Birth (also see Breech babies; Caesarean section; Cervix; Children; Contractions in Labor; Obstetrics; Postpartum period; Pregnancy; Reproductive system; Stillbirths; Umbilical cord; Uterus; Vagina), 61, 62, 73–90, 93, 125, 156, 219
Birth control pills, 108
Birth defects, 77
Bitter cucumber (see *Colocynthis*)
Black emancipation, 41
Black medical schools (also see Medical schools), 45
Black snakeroot (see *Actaea racemosa*)
Black sulphide of antimony (see *Antimonium crudum*)

Blackie, Dr. Margery, 235
Bladder, 78, 82, 86, 108, 110, 111, 115
Bliss, Dr. D. W., 39
Blisters, 181
Blood (also see Arteries; Capillaries; Hematoma; Hemorrhage; Veins), 5, 14, 35, 64, 86, 91, 93, 108, 113, 114, 115, 133, 140, 156, 178, 188, 204, 213
Bloodletting, 35, 36, 91, 92
Blood pressure, 76, 114, 156, 157, 188
Blue cohosh (see *Caulophyllum*)
Board of Experts, 127
Bodymind, xvi, 21, 66, 189
Bodymind types (also see Personality types; Typology), 18, 113, 192–197, 234
Body types (also see Personality types; Typology), 18
Boericke, Dr. William, 231
Boils (skin), 127
Bones, 92, 116, 143, 173, 181, 206, 213
Boneset (see *Eupatorium perfoliatum*)
Borland, Douglas, 84
Boston Female Medical College, 41
Bostonians, The, 42
Boston University, 41, 43
Bouton, Jim, 175, 176
Bovista (puffball), 87
Boyd, W. E., 64
Bradford, Dr. Thomas L., 126
Brain, 11, 13, 14, 25, 96, 100, 143, 156, 186–189
Brand, Stewart, 8
Brazil, 49, 50, 128
Breast-feeding (also see Lactation; Milk), 77, 78, 87, 88, 140
Breasts (also see Mastitis; Nipples), 79, 88, 108
Breathing (also see Asphyxiation; Asthma; Congestion; Decongestants; Inhalers; Lungs; Mouth; Nose; Phlegm; Skin), 5, 25, 86, 88, 93, 99, 104, 128, 131, 139, 140, 142, 143, 147
Breech babies (also see Birth), 82, 83
Britain/British, 29, 47, 48, 59, 62, 63, 64, 65, 84, 86, 91, 94, 128, 177, 244, 245, 249
British Cycling Federation, 177
British Homoeopathic Association, 245
British Homoeopathic Journal, 244
British Homoeopathy Research Group, 244
British Journal of Clinical Pharmacology, 59, 164
British Medical Association, 24
British Medical Journal, 48
British Royal Family, 3, 29, 41, 48, 220, 224
Bronchioles, 140
Bronchitis (also see Lungs), 26
Bryant, William Cullen, 40
Bryonia (wild hops), 60, 81, 87, 88, 98, 130, 178, 181
Burk, Dr. Dean, 207
Burnett, Dr. J. Compton, 164
Burns/Burning sensations, 59, 100, 110, 111, 144, 145, 154, 181, 214
Bushmaster snake, venom of (see *Lachesis*)

Cadmium, 131
Caesarean section (also see Birth), 75, 76, 77, 85
Calcarea carbonica (calcium carbonate), 96, 97, 118, 168
Calcarea phosphorica (calcium phosphate), 97, 134, 180
Calcium, 117, 204, 215
Calcium carbonate (see *Calcarea carbonica*)
Calcium sulphide (see *Hepar sulph*)
Calendula, 86, 181, 214
Calves (also see Legs)
Campbell, Anthony, 233
Camphora (camphor), 86, 129
Canadian Medical Association Journal, 76
Cancer (also see Leukemia), 6, 28, 62, 63, 108, 116, 153, 154, 157, 159, 161, 163, 207
Candida albicans (yeast), 64, 111, 121
Cannon, Walter B., 4
Cantharis (Spanish fly), 110, 111
Capillaries (also see Arteries; Blood; Veins), 140
Capra, Fritjof, 4
Carbo veg (vegetable charcoal), 86, 179
Caries (also see Dental problems)
Carlson, Rick, xvi
Carnegie Foundation, 44
Case histories, 11, 27
Case-taking (homeopathic), 24, 148

Cassette tapes, 237–238, 242
Catharsis, 198
Cathartics, 73
Cats, 56
Cattle, 56, 62
Caulophyllum (blue cohosh), 61, 62, 83, 84, 110
Causticum (Hahnemann's potassium hydrate), 131
Celandine (see *Chelidonium*)
Cells, 5, 13, 14, 64, 93, 133, 140, 143
Cellulose, 149
Cervix (also see Women's health), 83
Ceylon, 49
Chamomilla (chamomile), 96, 97, 98, 110, 127, 212, 213
Cheeks (also see Face), 97, 144
Chelidonium (celandine), 62, 87
Chemicals, xv, 5, 63, 64, 109, 139, 140, 142, 154
Chemistry/Chemists (also see Biochemistry; Physiochemistry), 11, 15, 34, 36, 45, 121
Chemotherapy, 154
Cherry laurel (see *Laurocerasus*)
Chest (also see Breasts; Ribs), 143
"Chi," 15
Chicken pox, 5, 100, 131
Chickens, 64, 128, 130
Childbirth (see Birth)
Children (also see Birth; Obstetrics; Pediatrics; Pregnancy; Toys), 5, 6, 57, 73, 74, 75, 77, 78, 85, 87, 91–106, 114, 120, 122, 123, 124, 125, 127, 128, 140, 149, 205, 211, 221
Children's Hospital of Pittsburgh (Pa.), 124
Chile, 49
China/Chinese, 15, 33
Chionanthus (fringe-tree), 87
Chiropractors, xx, 28, 50, 175, 180, 248
Chlamydia (also see Venereal diseases), 111
Chloride of potassium (see *Kali muriaticum*)
Cholera (also see Epidemics), 40, 42, 57, 125, 126, 129
Cholesterol, 62
Chondromalacia (see "Runners knee"), 179, 180
Chou, Jessica, 65
Chowka, Peter Barry, 154

Christian Science, 41
Chronic conditions (also see Acute conditions), xv, xvi, xvii, xviii, xx, 16, 19, 20, 21, 22, 26, 27, 35, 43, 49, 51, 58, 79, 80, 88, 100, 108, 111, 112, 121, 123, 127, 128, 129, 130, 131, 144, 145, 146, 153–171, 210, 240, 250, 251
Cigarettes (see Smoking)
Cimicifuga (see *Actaea racemosa*)
Cinchona (Peruvian bark), 34, 131
Clark, John, 234
Clergy, 41
Clinical effects, 55, 58, 65
Clothing, 102, 115, 117
Clotting (see Blood)
Cloves, 103
Club moss (see *Lycopodium*)
Cocaine (also see Narcotics), 132
Co-factors, 132, 133, 134
Coffea (coffee), 97, 142, 212, 213, 214
Colchicine, 6
Colchicum (meadow saffron), 80
Colds (see Common colds)
Cole, K. C., 13
Colfax, Schulyer, 39
Colic, 96, 97, 98
Colocynthis (bitter cucumber), 98, 110, 180
Colon, 5
Combination medicines, 22, 23, 60, 61, 84, 142
Common colds, 92, 93, 96, 102, 103, 104, 115, 129, 130
Complementary medicine (also see "Alternative medicine"), 48, 219, 224
"Complexes" (see Combination medicines)
Complexion (also see Face), 114, 193
Computers, xv, 10, 14
Congestion (also see Decongestants; Lungs; Nose), 88, 141
Conium (hemlock), 131
Connecticut Department of Health, 133
Constipation, xiii, 28, 79, 81, 82, 88, 96, 114, 158–159
Constitutional medicines (also see Acute medicines; Fundamental medicines), 19, 20, 21, 22, 79, 80, 81, 82, 83, 127, 147, 161, 214, 229, 234
"Consultation clause," 38, 39, 44

Contractions in labor (also see Birth), 76, 83, 84

Conventional medicine (also see "Alternative medicine"; Natural therapies; Physicians), xiv, xv, xvi, xviii, xix, xxi, xxii, 6, 7, 17, 18, 25, 27, 33, 35, 36, 37, 38, 39, 40, 41, 42, 43, 44, 45, 46, 47, 48, 49, 50, 55, 58, 61, 75, 77, 79, 82, 83, 85, 86, 87, 91, 92, 96, 98, 99, 101, 104, 107, 109, 111, 116, 122, 126, 127, 128, 129, 130, 135, 140, 141, 142, 143, 146, 147, 148, 153, 155, 156, 160, 164, 166, 190, 219, 222, 224, 232

Convulsions, 95, 96

Cook, Dr. Trevor, 233

Cooper, Dr. Jack, 196

Coronary bypass surgery (also see Heart), 156

Corticosteroids, 132, 133, 175, 191

Cortisone, 17, 98, 99, 133, 141, 147, 175, 191

Coughs (also see Whooping cough), 5, 21, 22, 93, 95, 100, 102, 103, 129, 140, 145

Coulter, Catherine, 20, 113, 192–193, 200

Coulter, Harris, 232, 233

Cousins, Norman, 223

Cowpox, 34, 35

Cox, Dr. Christopher C., 38, 39

Cramps (also see Pain), 79, 82, 109, 110, 168, 177, 180

Cravings, 19, 102, 114, 117, 148, 150

Creams, 147

Creativity, 102

Crews, Dr. Richard, 232

Crop production (also see Food), 15

Crotalus horridus (venom of the rattlesnake), 134, 135

Crying (see Weeping)

Cucumber (see Colocynthis)

Cullen, William, 34

Cummings, Stephen, 230, 240

Cuprum metallicum (copper), 180

Cuts, abrasions, 181

Cuttlefish (see Sepia)

Cybernetics, 14

Cyclosporin, 133, 135

Cystitis (see Bladder)

Cysts, 108, 161, 166

Cytomegaloviruses (also see Viruses), xv

Cytotoxic testing, 148

Daisy (see Bellis perrenis)

Dangers of homeopathy (see Risks of homeopathy)

Dartmouth Medical College, 36

Davey, Dr. Ronald, 223–224

Davidson, Robert, 86

Davis, Nathan Smith, 36

Day, Christopher, 62

Deadly nightshade (see Belladonna)

Death (also see Mortality rates; Murder; Suicide), 16, 25, 40, 42, 43, 86, 91, 93, 96, 155, 156

Decongestants (also see congestion), 93, 141

Defense system (also see Immune system), xiii, xvii, xviii, xix, xx, xxiii, 3, 4, 5, 8, 9, 14, 16, 21, 22, 29, 66, 77, 92, 93, 96, 97, 98, 112, 119, 122, 128, 132, 135, 140, 147, 158–163, 191–192, 200, 220, 221

Delgado, José, 13

Delphic Oracle, 7

Democritus, 190

Dental problems/Dentistry/Dentists (also see American Dental Association; Calcium; Caries; Eating; Extraction of teeth; Food; Gingivitis; Gums; Mouth; Peridontal disease; Plaque; Sugar; Teething; TMJ syndrome), xx, 50, 60, 92, 168, 203–218, 235, 245

Dentures, 203, 214

Dependency, 143

Depression, psychological (also see Antidepressants; Emotions), 9, 188, 189, 190, 191

Descartes, 158

Desensitization shots (see Injections)

Detoxification (also see Toxicity; Toxicology), 77

Development (see Growth and development)

Dhawale, Dr. M. L., 234

Diabetes/Diabetics, 166

Diagnosis, xvi, xvii, xx, 24, 28, 102, 109, 111, 114, 115, 121, 124, 129, 134, 139, 148, 150

Diarrhea, 5, 81, 96, 133, 207, 211

Diastase, 64

Dickens, Charles, 41
Diet, 25, 62, 79, 117, 148, 149, 150, 206
Digestion (also see Defecation; Eating; Food; Indigestion; Intestines; Mouth; Stomach), 120, 128, 139, 140, 147, 149, 150, 151
Digitalis, 6
Dilation, 140
Dilution (of medicines), 12, 13, 15, 28, 47, 57
Diphtheria, 100
Discharges (also see Fluids; Pus), 5, 88, 93, 104, 115, 131, 144
Disease (also see Bacteria; Germs; Viruses), xiv, xv, xvi, xvii, xviii, xix, xx, xxi, xxiii, 3, 4, 6, 9, 10, 16, 17, 18, 19, 22, 24, 27, 28, 35, 37, 42, 43, 45, 46, 55, 57, 60, 73, 76, 78, 87, 98, 99, 100, 108, 109, 111, 112, 115, 119–138, 139, 140, 141, 142, 143, 147, 153–171, 187
Disposition, 18
Disraeli, Benjamin, 41
District of Columbia, 38
Diuretics, 109
Diverticulosis, 159
Dizziness (see Vertigo)
DNA (Deoxyribonucleic acid), 13, 161, 205
Doctors (see Physicians)
Doctrine of Signatures, 7, 30
Dogs, 56
Dog's milk (see *Lac caninum*)
Double-bind (see Therapeutic double-bind), 198
Double-blind studies (also see Experimentation), 55, 56, 58, 59, 60, 61, 62, 84, 117, 146, 164, 213
Dowsing, 24
Dreams (also see Hallucinations; Sleep), 95, 166
Drink (also see Food; Thirst), 8, 95, 102, 113
Drooling, 96, 97
Drowsiness (also see Sleep), 141, 149
Drug companies, 37, 46
Drug provings, 9, 10, 26, 27, 28, 30, 57, 222, 224
Dryness, 95, 113, 115, 116, 143
Dry socket, 214
Dubos, René, xix, 126, 223

Ducks, 130

Ears/Earaches (also see Mastoiditis; otitis media), 100, 122, 123, 125, 131, 212, 213, 215
East Germany (see Germany)
Eastman, Zabina, 41
Eating (also see Diet; Digestion; Drink; Fasting; Food; Indigestion; Mouth; Throat), 80, 101, 103, 113, 114, 115, 145, 146, 147, 149, 150
Ecology, 119, 122, 132, 135, 148
Economics, 37, 45
Ecosystems, 66
Eczema (also see Allergies; Skin), 96, 98, 99, 139, 147, 150
Eddy, Mary Baker, 41
Einstein, Albert, 189
Eizayaga, Dr. Francisco X., 18, 19, 49
Elderly (see old age)
Electroacupuncture machines, 23–24, 210
Electromagnetic signals, 13
Electronics, 23
Embryos, 64, 128
Elimination diet (also see Diet), 150
Emergencies, 25, 73, 154
Emotional symptoms (see Symptoms)
Emotions (also see Anger; Depression; Fear; Grief; Hatred; Hysteria; Lethargy; Moodiness; Nervousness; Tranquilizers), xiv, 3, 5, 16, 19, 22, 81, 97, 98, 99, 103, 112, 113, 156, 164, 173, 190
Endorphins, 63
Energy, 13, 19, 28, 100, 102, 114, 117
England/Englishmen (see Britain/British)
Environment, 25, 26, 27, 62, 79, 102, 120, 135, 139, 165, 167, 190, 197
Enzymes, 11, 64, 87
Ephedrine, 142
Epidemics (also see Cholera; Plague; Polio; Scarlet fever; Typhoid fever; Yellow fever), xiv, xix, 40, 42, 43, 57, 126, 134, 164
Epidemiology/Epidemiologists, 126, 132
Epilepsy/Epileptics, 96, 166
Episiotomies (also see Birth), 75, 76, 85
Epstein-Barr virus (also see Viruses), xv, 130
Erickson, Milton, 198

"Essence" of symptoms (also see Symptoms), 19
Estrogen, 108, 116, 117
Ethical codes, 38
Eupatorium perfoliatum (boneset), 130
Euphrasia (eyebright), 130, 144
Exercise, xiv, 114, 145, 156
Exhaustion (also see Weakness), 85, 102, 115, 156, 158
Experimentation (also see Double-blind studies; Drug provings), 37, 55, 56, 119
Externalization (of disease), 17
Extraction of teeth (also see Dental problems), 60
Eyebright (see *Euphrasia*)
Eyes (also see Face), 7, 139, 144, 145

Face (also see Cheeks; Complexion; Ears; Eyes; Lips; Mouth; Nose), 76, 84, 86, 88, 95, 115
Faculty of Homoeopathy, 244, 249
Faith healing, xvi
Farmers, 120
Fastidiousness (see Perfectionism)
Fasting (also see Eating), 115
Fatigue (see Exhaustion)
Faust, 7
FDA Consumer (also see Food and Drug Administration), 50
Fear (also see Emotions), 16, 28, 86, 95, 97, 102, 113, 156, 186, 190, 193, 198, 211
Female emancipation, 41
Fenoprofen, 61
Ferdinand, Grand Duke, 35
Ferrum phos (phosphate of iron), 127, 129
Fertilizers, 15, 65
Fetal distress syndrome, 75
Fetuses (also see Birth), 75, 76, 77, 78, 81, 82, 93
Fever (also see Rheumatic fever; Scarlet fever; Yellow fever), 4, 5, 17, 34, 57, 73, 86, 88, 93, 94, 95, 96, 97, 123, 129, 133
Fibroids (see Tumors)
Fibrosarcoma, 63
Fibrositis, 60, 165
Fillings, dental, 208–211
Fingers, 97
Fischer, Dr. Richard, 213

Fitness (see physical fitness)
Fleming, Alexander, 121
Flexibility
Flexner, Abraham, 44
Flexner Report, 44, 45
Flick, Bart, 178
Flu (see Influenza)
Fluids (also see Discharges; Water), 123
Fluorescent lights, 87
Fluoride/Fluoridation, 204–211
Flushing (also see Redness), 84, 95, 113, 116
Food (also see Allergies; Breast-feeding; Crop production; Diet; Digestion; Drink; Eating; Health food stores; Hunger; Indigestion; Intestines; Nutrition; Stomach), xv, 8, 11, 19, 26, 80, 81, 85, 98, 113, 125, 133, 139, 147, 148, 149, 150
Food and Drug Administration (FDA), 77, 92, 155
"Force, The," 15
Forceps (also see Birth), 75, 76
Foundation for Homeopathic Education and Research, 70, 243
Fractures, 180
France/Frenchmen, 35, 39, 48, 61, 63, 79, 84, 87, 130, 145, 206
Freshwater sponge (see *Badiaga*)
Freud, Sigmund, 199
Fringe-tree (see *Chionanthus*)
Frost, Robert, 224
Functional disturbances, 158–159
Fundamental medicines (also see Constitutional medicines), 19, 20, 80
Futurists, xv, xvi

Gallo, Dr. Robert, 134
Gandhi, Mahatma, 3, 29, 49
Gardnerella (Hemophilus), 111
Garlic (also see Food), 103
Garrison, William Lloyd, 41
Gas (see Abdominal gas)
Gastroenteritis (also see Intestines; Stomach), 129
Gates, Frederick, 45, 46
Gelb, Dr. Harold, 215
Gelsemium (yellow jasmine), 61, 84, 130, 131, 211
Gemmell, Dr. David, 230
Genetics (also see Predispositions), 19,

77, 79, 99, 132, 160
George, Dr. John, 83, 85
Geothermal changes, 11
German measles, 100
German viper (see *Vipera*)
Germany/Germans, 34, 35, 60, 62, 73, 79
Germination (also see Seeds), 64
Germs (also see Bacteria; Disease; Viruses), 74, 119, 121, 122, 215
Gestalt therapy, 199
Gibson, Dr. D. M., 20, 231, 234
Gilbert, Walter, 121
Gingivitis (also see Dental problems; Gums), 204
Glasgow Homeopathic Hospital, 59, 146
Goethe, Johann Wolfgang, 7, 41
Golas, Natalie, 150
Golbitz, Frances Golos, 150
Gold salts, 6
Gonorrhea (also see Venereal diseases), 121, 160–161
Gout, 6
Graedon, Joe, 141, 209
Gram, Hans, 37
Graphities (graphite), 118, 127
Grass, 141, 146
Great Britain (see Britain/British)
Greece/Greeks, 33, 50
Greek mythology, 7
Greeley, Horace, 40
Greenberg, Dr. D. S., 154
Grief (also see Emotions), 114, 115
Grossinger, Richard, 233
Growth and development, 92, 99, 101, 120, 128
Gums (also see Dental problems; Peridontal disease), 97, 204, 212, 214, 215
Gutmann, Dr. Viktor, 233
Gynecology/Gynecologists (also see Women's health), 73, 83, 108

Hahnemann, Dr. Samuel, 6, 29, 33, 34, 35, 37, 42, 46, 47, 160, 162, 185, 230, 232, 251
Hahnemann Medical Clinic, 246
Hahnemann Medical College, 43
Hahnemann Society, 29
Hahnemann's calcium sulphide (see *Hepar sulph*)

Hahnemann's potassium hydrate (see *Causticum*)
Haiti, 132
Hallucinations, 95, 101
Hamamelis (witch hazel), 82
Harper's Magazine, 40
Harvard University, 36, 41, 121
Hatred (also see Emotions), 115, 117
Hawthorne, Nathaniel, 40
Hay Fever (also see Allergies), 22, 59, 139, 146, 150, 165, 206, 213, 215
Headaches, xiii, 9, 10, 17, 19, 26, 28, 46, 88, 101, 102, 110, 114, 115, 117, 139, 151, 190, 219
Healing, xiv, xvi, xvii, xx, xxi, xxiii, 3, 4, 7, 8, 15, 16, 17, 18, 20, 23, 25, 29, 30, 33, 40, 49, 57, 66, 78, 82, 86, 93, 94, 96, 104, 112, 122, 135, 158, 189
Healing crises, 20, 58
Health food stores, 22
Hearing, 215
Heart/Heart conditions, 6, 16, 117, 130, 142, 155, 156, 157, 173, 181, 188, 196, 235
Heat (also see Coldness; Temperature), 84, 86, 88, 95, 97, 102, 103, 110, 114, 115, 116, 117, 144, 145
Heightened awareness, xvi
Heimlich, Jane, 230
Helleborus (snow-rose), 96
Hematoma (also see Blood), 86, 178
Hemlock (see *Conium*)
Hemophilus (see *Gardnerella*)
Hemorrhage (also see Blood), 76, 213
Hemorrhoids, 79, 82, 159
Hepar sulph (Hahnemann's calcium sulphide), 101, 127, 212, 214
Hepatitis (also see Liver), 129
Herbs/Herbalists, 7, 34, 36, 94
Heredity, xviii, 119, 160–162
Hering, Dr. Constantine, 6, 16, 17
"Hering's Law of Cure," 17, 18, 26, 147, 200, 223
Herpes, 78, 82, 128, 130, 133
High-tech medicine, xvi
"High-touch" medicine, xvi
Hippocrates, 7, 22, 30, 33, 232
Histamine (also see Antihistamines), 64, 140, 145
HIV (see Human Immunodeficiency Virus)

Hives (also see Allergies), 139, 145, 146
Hjermann, Dr. I., 157
Hole, Dr. Ben, 130
Holistic medicine, xvi, 18
Holland (see Netherlands)
Homeopathic books, 79
Homeopathic case-taking (see Case-taking)
Homeopathic colleges, 40, 41, 43, 44, 45, 47, 49, 50, 210, 236
Homeopathic Educational Services, 31, 70, 231, 237, 238, 240, 242, 248
Homeopathic journals, 43
Homeopathic medicine kits, 242, 250
Homeopathic organizations, 242–245
Homeopathic pharmacies (also see Pharmacists), 242
Homeopathic repertories (see Repertories)
Homeopathic research (see Research)
Homeopathic study groups (231, 236–240)
Homeopathic training programs, 243–247
Homeostasis, xix, xx, 4, 158
Homoeopathic Medical Research Council, 244
Homosexuality/Homosexuals, 133
Hops, wild (see *Bryonia*)
Hormones, 108, 109, 110, 114, 116, 176, 188, 204
Horses, 56
Hospices, 219
Hospitals, 25, 40, 42, 47, 59, 74, 75, 87, 92, 124, 146, 154, 155, 219
Hospital Ste. Marguerite, 39
Host resistance, 119, 122
Hubbard, Elizabeth Wright, 118, 232
Hughes, Dr. Richard, 235
Human Immunodeficiency Virus (HIV), 134
Human Toxicology, 62
Humanistic psychology, 222
Hunger (also see Food), 81
Hygiene, 125, 132, 203, 215
Hyperactivity (also see Underactivity), 6, 22, 23, 100, 101, 102, 196
Hypericum (St. John's wort), 60, 63, 131, 180, 213
Hyperirritability (see Irritation)
Hypersensitivity (also see Allergies; Sensitivity), 13, 14, 102, 115, 139,
140, 149, 150, 167, 187, 193, 206, 207, 210, 212, 214
Hypertension, 142, 155
Hyperthyroidism (also see Thyroid gland), 115
Hypnosis, 48, 175
Hypoadrenalism (also see Adrenal gland), 115
Hypochondriacs, 193
Hypoinsulinism (also see Insulin), 115
Hysteria (also see Emotions), 85
Iatrogenic (doctor-induced) conditions, xix, 134, 155, 221
Idiosyncrasies, 11, 21, 37, 115, 139
Imberechts, Dr. Jacques, 82, 84
"Immune overload hypothesis," 132
Immune system (also see Defense system), xiii, xiv, xvii, xviii, xix, xx, xxiii, 3, 5, 9, 14, 22, 29, 64, 66, 77, 92, 93, 112, 119, 120, 122, 124, 132, 134, 135, 139, 140, 164–165, 206, 209, 220, 221
Immunization (also see Vaccines), 6, 35, 100, 128
Immunology (also see Psychoneuroimmunology), 6, 14, 59, 64, 94, 124, 140, 210
Immunosuppression, 132, 133, 135
Impotence (sexual), 156
Incubation (also see Birth), 87
India, 14, 33, 34, 49, 62
Indigestion (also see Digestion), 9, 26, 28, 46, 80, 81, 92, 97, 98, 101, 102, 104
Individualization (of homeopathic treatment/doses), 9, 11, 22, 25, 28, 45, 60, 61, 79, 80, 103, 109, 112, 118, 130, 131, 135, 144, 147, 168, 190, 197, 211, 221, 222, 249
Infants (see Birth; Children)
Infection, xv, xvi, xviii, xix, xx, 4, 5, 7, 25, 43, 49, 57, 64, 74, 78, 79, 82, 86, 93, 94, 96, 100, 108, 110, 111, 112, 119–138, 155, 158, 159
Inflammation, 5, 23, 61, 87, 91, 94, 97, 111, 140, 141, 175
Influenza (also see Lungs), 5, 126, 129, 130, 131
Inhalers, 143
Injuries (also see Stress), 85, 86, 100, 173–183, 231
Insects, 142

Insecticides (also see Pest control), 120
Insomnia (also see Sleep), 10, 22, 57, 78, 82, 101, 102, 193, 212
Institute for Complementary Medicine, 220
Insulin, 115, 186
Insurance companies, 43, 74, 129, 219
Interferon, 5, 93
International Foundation for Homeopathy, 243
International Journal of Immunotherapy, 64
Intestines (also see Gastroenteritis), 119
Ions (also see Atoms; Molecules; Protons; Subatomic activity), 11
Ipecacuanha (Ipecac), 80
Iridology, 148
Iron (also see *Ferrum phos*), 25, 26
Irritation/Irritants/Irritability (also see Emotions), xiii, 16, 17, 21, 28, 79, 81, 82, 84, 97, 98, 104, 110, 114, 115, 117, 121, 133, 140, 144
Italy/Italians, 50
Itching, 100, 121
Jackson, Dr. Douglas, 174
James, Henry, 42
James, William, 40
Jantsch, Erich, 4
Jasmine (see *Gelsemium*)
Jaundice, 86, 87
Jenkins, Michael, 64, 65
Jenner, Edward, 34, 35
John Bastyr College of Naturopathic Medicine, 246
Johns Hopkins University, 41
Johnson, Andrew, 39
Joints (of the body), 17
Jones, Raynor, 64, 65
Jouanny, Dr. Jacque, 235
Journal of Dental Research, 206
Journalists, 132
Journal of the American Institute of Homeopathy, 65
Journal of the American Medical Association (JAMA), 155
Jungian psychology, 192, 199, 233, 234

Kali bichromicum (bichromate of potash), 59, 131
Kali carbonicum (potassium carbonate), 131
Kali iodatum (potassium iodide), 131

Kali muriaticum (chloride of potassium), 131
Kali sulphuricum (potassium sulphate), 131
Kalmia (mountain laurel), 131
Kant, Immanuel, 187
Kay, Alan, xxiii
Kent, James Tyler, 14, 20, 162, 230, 234, 235
Kepler, Johannes, 14
"Ki," 15
Kidneys, 77, 166
Kinesiology (see Applied kinesiology), 24
Kluger, Matthew, 4
Knees (also see Legs)
Koehler, Dr. Gerhard, 232
Kraus, Dr. Hans, 181

Labor (see Birth)
Lac caninum (dog's milk), 87, 88
Lacerations, 76
Lachesis (venom of the bushmaster snake), 110, 117, 127, 134, 213
Lactation (also see Breast-feeding; Milk), 77
Lancet, 56, 59, 91, 146, 157
Lancets, 91
Lappé, Marc, 121
Lasers, 141
"Law of Similars," 6, 7, 8, 9, 11, 13, 14, 19, 30, 33, 34, 101
Laurocerasus (cherry laurel), 86
Lawrence, Dr. Ronald, 176
Lead, 36
"Learning disability" (see Hyperactivity)
Ledum (marsh tea), 177, 214
Leeches, 35, 36
Legs (also see Ankles; Calves; Feet; Knees; Thighs; Toes), 79, 82, 86, 103, 168, 177, 179
Lessell, Dr. Colin, 235
LeShan, Lawrence, 190
Lethargy (also see Emotions), 81, 95, 104
Leukemia (also see Blood; Cancer), 91, 157
Leukotienes, 140
Levin, Alan Scott, 150
Librium, 156
Licensing examinations (see Medical

board examinations)
Life expectancy, 125
"Life force" (see "Vital force")
Life insurance companies (see Insurance companies)
Lifestyle, 25, 27, 79, 117, 165
Ligaments, 204
Lignin, 149
Ligament injury, 178
Limits of homeopathy, 24–28
Lincoln, Abraham, 38
Lips (also see Face; Mouth), 88, 144
Liquorice, wild (see Sarsaparilla)
Lister, Dr. Joseph, 94
Lithotomy position (also see Birth), 76
Little, Sally, 175
Liver (also see Hepatitis), 77, 87, 92, 130
Lobotomy, 186
Longfellow, Henry Wadsworth, 40
Luce, Gay Gaer, xxi
Lungs (also see Breathing; Bronchitis; Congestion; Influenza; Pneumonia; Tuberculosis; Whooping cough), 99, 143, 156
Lycopodium (club moss), 87, 98

MacAdoo, Bob, 175
Macrophages, 64
Magic, 7
Magnesia phosphorica/Mag phos (phosphate of magnesia), 98, 110, 131, 180
Magnetic resonance imaging (see Nuclear magnetic resonance)
Magnets, 7
Malaria, 34
Malnutrition (see Nutrition)
Marathons, 177
Marijuana, 132
Marrow (see Bones)
Maslow, Abraham, 222
Martial arts, 8
Mast cells (also see Cells), 140
Mastitis (also see Breasts; Inflammation), 56, 62, 87, 88
Mastoiditis (also see Ears), 123
Materia medicas, 10, 20, 36, 81, 142, 163, 193, 215, 231, 234–235, 236, 238
Maxmen, Dr. Jerrold, 187
Mayans, 33

Mayo Clinic, 130
Meadow saffron (see Colchicum)
Measles, 100
Medical board examinations, 43, 44, 45
"Medical chauvinism," xxi
Medical checkups, 173
Medical education, 36, 40
Medical emergencies (see Emergencies)
Medical Forum, 209
Medical journals, 39, 46, 47, 56, 91, 146, 155
Medical jurisprudence, 36
Medical malpractice suits, 74
Medical philosophy, xix, 8, 37
Medical schools (also see Black medical schools; Homeopathic colleges), 40, 43, 44, 45, 48, 50, 64
Medical societies, 38, 40, 47
Meditation, xvi
Mendelsohn, Dr. Robert, 87, 97
Meningitis, 25, 91, 95, 128
Meningococcin, 128
Menninger, Charles Frederick, 185, 189
Menopause (also see Women's health), 108, 116, 117, 118, 204
Menstruation (also see Women's health), 10, 19, 108, 113, 115, 116, 204
Mental illness, xv, 17, 185–202
Mental symptoms (see Symptoms)
Menuhin, Yehudi, 3, 29, 51, 244
Mercuric bichloride, 74
Mercuric chloride, 64
Mercurius (mercury), 36, 100, 111, 127, 131, 134, 160, 211, 212, 213
Mercury fillings (see Amalgam fillings)
Methylphenidate (see Ritalin)
Mexico, 50
Mezereum (spurge olive), 131
Miasm, 160–162
Mice, 63, 64
Microbes, xix
Microbiology/Microbiologists (also see Biology), 126
Microdoses (of homeopathic medicines), xvii, 6, 7, 8, 9, 10, 11, 12, 14, 15, 22, 25, 27, 34, 40, 50, 55, 56, 57, 58, 62, 63, 64, 66, 80, 83, 100, 111, 128, 130, 131, 135, 142, 145, 146, 147, 190, 222, 233
Microorganisms (also see Organisms),

111, 112, 119, 122
Middletown Asylum for the Insane (see
State Homeopathic Hospital, at Mid-
dletown), 197
Midwifery/Midwives (also see Obste-
trics), 36, 73, 78, 81
Milk (also see Breast-feeding; Food;
Lac caninum; Lactation), 38, 77, 87,
93, 98, 102, 140, 150, 206
Mind-altering drugs, 107
"Minimal brain damage" (see Hyper-
activity)
Missionaries, 115
Mitterrand, François, 48
Molds, (organic), 64, 139, 141
Molecules (also see Atoms; Ions; Pro-
tons; Subatomic activity), 13, 15, 57
Mollusks (also see Food), 113, 114
Monkshood (see *Aconite*)
Moodiness (also see Emotions), 81, 113,
186
Moore, Sherrie, 181
Morning sickness, 80, 81
Morphine, 61, 62, 63, 73
Mortality rates (also see Death), 40, 42,
43, 73, 74, 76, 77, 125, 126
Moskowitz, Dr. Richard, 82
Mosquitoes, 120
Motor defects, 96
Mottling of the teeth, 205, 206
Mountain daisy (see *Arnica*)
Mountain laurel (see *Kalmia*)
Mouth (also see Dental problems; Face;
Lips), 81, 95, 97, 113, 115, 203–218
Mucus/Mucous membranes, 5, 84, 93,
115, 141, 143
Mumps, 100, 131
Murder (also see Death),
Muscles, 24, 82, 83, 85, 93, 95, 109,
142, 148, 173, 175, 177, 181, 207
Music, 12, 13
Mussels (also see Food), 114
Mustard gas, 59

Nader, Ralph, 208
Naloxone, 63
Napoleonic Wars, 35
Narcotics, 132
National Bureau of Standards, 15
National Cancer Institute, 153, 154,
207
National Center for Health Statistics,
155
National Center for Homeopathy, 231,
232, 243, 246, 248
National College of Naturopathic Medi-
cines, 246
National Institute of Health, 224
National Institute of Mental Health,
186
Native American Indians, 33
Natrum mur (salt [sodium chloride]),
19, 110, 112, 114, 115, 117, 130, 134
Natrum sulph (sodium sulphate), 87
Natural therapies (also see "Alternative
medicine"; Conventional medicine),
xiv, xv, xx, 122, 148
Nature, Natural law, 9, 14, 15, 66,
164, 188, 223, 224, 246
Nature, 207
Naturopaths, xx, 18, 50, 175, 246, 247
Nausea, 60, 78, 80, 81, 82, 103
Neisseria meningitidis (also see Men-
ingitis), 128
Nerves/Nervous system, 76, 93, 108,
128, 133, 187, 235
Nervousness (also see Emotions), 22,
84, 101, 193
Neumann, Hans H., 133
Neuralgia, 60, 131, 213
Neurology/Neurologists, xvi, 5, 13, 56,
57, 93, 188
Netherlands/Dutchmen, 37, 49, 75
Neurotransmitters, 187
Neustaedter, Randall, 127
New England Female Medical College,
41
New England Journal of Medicine,
122, 124, 133, 153, 154, 155, 207
New Scientist, 205
Newsweek, 132
New York City, 118
New York Homeopathic Society, 40
New York State, 41
New York State Medical Society, 38
New York Times, 48
Nigeria, 50
Nitricum acid (nitric acid), 134
Nitroglycerine, 6
"Nonspecific" illness, xvii
Nose (also see Face), 93, 103, 131, 139,
141, 144, 145
Nouvel Observateur, Le, 48

Nuclear magnetic resonance (NMR), 63
Nuclear radiation (see Radiation)
Nurses, xx, 50, 74, 78, 96
Nursing (see Breast-feeding)
Nutrition/Nutrients (also see Food), xiv, xvi, 25, 81, 87, 93, 119, 120, 125, 132, 157, 204, 219
Nux vomica (poison nut), 21, 80, 81, 87, 96, 98, 101, 111, 131, 179, 192, 194–196
Oats (see *Avena sativa*)
Obstetrics/Obstetricians (also see Birth; Children; Midwifery), xx, 73, 74, 75, 79, 82, 83, 88
Office of Technology Assessment, 58, 221
Old age, 149, 156, 188, 214
Old people's homes, 40
Opium, 86, 96
Organisms (also see Microorganisms), 14, 15, 16, 19, 28, 29, 65, 66, 74, 79, 96, 111, 123, 124, 147, 148, 150
Orphan asylums, 40
Orth, Maureen, 29
Orthodox medicine (see Conventional medicine)
Orthopedic surgery/surgeons, 174
Oscillococcinum, 130
Osler, Sir William, 55, 112
Osteoarthritis (see Arthritis)
Osteopathy, osteopaths, 180, 219, 245
Osteoporosis (also see Bones), 116
Otitis media (also see Ears), 122, 123
Ovaries, 108, 116
Overdoses (see Toxic), 5, 27, 80, 133, 143, 147, 163, 206
Overexertion (see Exhaustion)
Overreactions (see Hypersensitivity)
Overweight, 168
Pagliano, Dr. John, 174
Pain (also see Cramps; Injuries; Stress; Trauma), 7, 8, 27, 28, 60, 61, 63, 73, 76, 78, 81, 82, 83, 85, 88, 96, 98, 100, 102, 103, 104, 109, 110, 111, 114, 115, 129, 145, 155, 156, 158
Painkillers, 174
Pakistan, 49
Palpitations (also see Heart), 117
Pancreatitis, 28
Panos, Dr. Maesimund, 230
Paracelsus, 7, 33, 232, 234
"Paradoxical action" (of drugs), 101

"Paradoxical intention," 198
Parasites, 133
Parathyroid gland, 204, 215
Paris Academy, 39
Parotidinum (also see Mumps), 131
Parsons, Dr. Philip, 213
Pasteur, Louis, 119, 122
Pathogens, 5, 128
Pathology, 5, 19, 27, 36, 44, 45, 108
Patterns, 13, 17, 18, 19, 21, 28, 83, 102, 115, 143
Peak performance, 173–183
Peck, Jonathan, xvi
Pediatrics/Pediatricians (also see Children), xx, 57, 75, 87, 91–106
Pendulums, 24
Penicillin, 64, 121, 132, 133
Penis, 133
People's Pharmacy, The, 141
Peridontal disease (also see Dental problems), 204
Perineum (also see Birth), 76, 86
Periosteum, 179, 213
Personality types (also see Body types; Bodymind Types; Typology), 18, 192–197
Perspiration, 17, 19, 95, 115, 116
Pest control (also see Insecticides), 125
Pharmacists/Pharmacies/Pharmacology (also see Homeopathic Pharmacies; Pharmacology journals, Pharmacy schools; Prescriptions), xvii, xviii, xxiii, 6, 11, 12, 14, 33, 34, 35, 38, 40, 44, 48, 50, 55, 58, 59, 121, 245
Pharmacology journals, 60, 64
Pharmacy schools, 48, 63
Pheromones, 14
Phlegm (also see Breathing), 86
Phobias (see Fear)
Phosphate of iron (see *Ferrum phos*)
Phosphate of magnesia (see *Magnesia phosphorica*)
Phosphoricum acidum (phosphoric acid), 131
Phosphorus, 19, 21, 101, 118, 130, 134, 213
Physical fitness, xvi, 157, 173, 219
Physical symptoms (see Symptoms)
Physical therapy, 18, 175, 180
Physician assistants, xx, 50
Physicians (also see Conventional medi-

cine; Women physicians), xv, xvi, xvii, xx, xxi, xxii, xxiii, 4, 5, 34, 38, 41, 47, 48, 49, 50, 55, 56, 60, 73, 74, 76, 77, 78, 83, 87, 92, 96, 101, 107, 109, 115, 116, 120, 123, 128, 129, 141, 142, 143, 148, 154, 155, 156, 187, 219, 223

Physicians' Desk Reference, 155, 206

Physics/Physicists, 4, 7, 13, 14

Physiology/Physiologists, xvi, xvii, xxii, 4, 14, 36, 45, 66, 87, 93, 94, 122, 123, 143, 147

Phytolacca (pokeroot), 87, 127

Pigs, 62, 84

Pitcairn, Richard, 247

Pius X, Pope, 41

Placebos, 17, 44, 55, 56, 57, 58, 59, 60, 61, 62, 63, 84, 123, 125, 146

Plague (also see Epidemics), 125

Plantarfasciitis, 178

Plantago (plantain), 213

Plants, xvii, 5, 66, 139

Plaque (also see Dental problems), 204

"Pluralism," 23

Pneumonia (also see Lungs), 122, 126

Podiatry/Podiatrists, 50, 181

Poison ivy (see *Rhus tox*)

Poison nut (see *Nux vomica*)

Pokeroot (see *Phytolacca*)

Polio (also see Epidemics), 126

Pollen, 59, 64, 139, 141, 146

Postpartum period (also see Birth), 78, 80, 88

Potassium, 109

Potassium carbonate (see *Kali carbonicum*)

Potassium hydrate (see *Causticum*)

Potassium iodide (see *Kali iodatum*)

Potassium sulphate (see *Kali sulphuricum*)

Potency/Potentization (of homeopathic doses), 9, 11, 14, 20, 22, 23, 26, 27, 28, 46, 47, 57, 58, 62, 63, 65, 83, 131, 135, 141, 146, 211, 224

"Prana," 15

Predispositions (also see Genetics, Hereditary, Miasm), 122, 132

Pregnancy (also see Birth), 61, 73–90, 92, 93, 204

Premenstrual syndrome (PMS), 108, 109, 110, 115

Prescriptions (also see Pharmacists), xv, 6, 10, 18, 19, 20, 21, 28, 29, 46, 51, 57, 60, 77, 79, 80, 83, 85, 86, 107, 108, 109, 112, 115, 116, 120, 124, 125, 127, 129, 130, 131, 142, 143, 147, 156, 164

Presley, Elvis, xiii

Prigogine, Ilya

Prince Charles (see also Britain's Royal Family), 220

Prison, 196

Progesterone, 108, 116

Progestin, 116, 117

Prophylaxis, 128, 129

Propranolol (Inderal), 156

Prostaglandins, 109, 110

Prostate, 142

Protein, 15, 93

Protons (also see Atoms; Ions; Molecules; Subatomic activity), 63

Provings (see Drug provings)

Psora, 160

Psorinum, 118

Psychiatry/Psychiatrists, xvi

Psychoanalysis/Psychoanalysts, 198, 200

Psychoneuroimmunology (also see Immunology), xvi

Psychological symptoms (see Symptoms)

Psychology/Psychologists, xiv, xvi, xx, xxii, 11, 18, 19, 20, 21, 50, 56, 78, 87, 102, 104, 107, 109, 110, 112, 114, 117, 119, 140, 143, 147, 148, 149, 185–202, 219, 222, 248

Psychosocial, 187

Psychotherapy, 18

Puberty, 204

Puffball (see *Bovista*)

Pulsatilla (windflower), 21, 61, 65, 80, 81, 82, 84, 98, 100, 110, 111, 112, 113, 127, 131

Punctures, 214

Pus (also see Discharges), 88, 123

Pyrogen (artificial sepsin), 214

Quinine, 73

Rabbits, 62

Radiation, 6, 77

Radionics, 24

Rape, 196

Rashes, 16, 17, 26, 96, 101, 133

Rats, 62
Rattlesnake, venom of (see *Crotalus horridus*)
"Rebound effect," 98, 141, 160
Recreational drug use, 132, 133
Rectal intercourse, 132
Redness (also see Flushing), 95, 97, 144
Reeve, Christopher, 42
Reeves, Whit, 177
Regeneration, 14, 66
Reich, Wilhelm, 199
Reilly, Pat, 175
Relaxation, xvi, 219
Religion, xvi, 115
Renner, Dr. John, 81
Repertories, 10, 231, 236
Reproductive system (also see Birth), 108
Resch, Dr. Gerhard, 233
Research, 55–70, 123, 124, 128, 134, 135, 140, 143, 145, 146, 150, 153, 163, 213, 220, 222, 223, 233, 244, 245
Research Council for Complementary Medicine, 220
Resonance, 13, 15
Restlessness, 95, 102, 103, 104
Revere, Paul, 203
Reyes Syndrome, 5, 93
Rheumatic fever, 123, 124
Rheumatism, 60
Rheumatoid arthritis (see Arthritis)
Rhododendron, 179
Rhus tox (poison ivy), 59, 61, 100, 127, 130, 178, 179, 180
Ribs (also see Chest), 181
RICE treatment, 174
Ries, Dr. Stanley, 15
Ringer, Sidney, 94
Risks of homeopathy, 24–28
Ritalin (methylphenidate), 6, 101
Roberts, H. A., 232
Rockefeller, John D., Sr., 3, 29, 40, 45, 46
Romeo and Juliet, 7
Rubsamen, Dr. David, 74
"Runner's knee" (Chondromalacia), 179
Ruta (rue), 213, 214
Rush, Dr. Benjamin, 35, 91, 92
Russians (see also Soviet Union), 15
Ruta (rue), 179, 180

St. John's wort (see *Hypericum*)
Salivary glands, 204, 215
Salk, Dr. Jonas, 122
Salt (see *Natrum mur*)
Salvia (sage), 212, 214
San Martín, José de, 49
Sarsaparilla (wild liquorice), 111
Savage, Dr. Richard, 128
Scarlet fever (also see Epidemics), 57, 125, 129
Schizophrenia, 16, 186, 187
Schmidt, Kate, 176
Sciatica, 180
Science/Scientists, xiv, xvi, xvii, xviii, xx, xxii, xxiii, 3, 6, 7, 10, 11, 13, 14, 15, 19, 28, 29, 34, 35, 36, 37, 40, 42, 44, 45, 55, 56, 62, 63, 64, 65, 66, 121, 122, 125, 128, 132, 140, 142, 164–165, 206, 221, 222, 223
Science, 204
Scientific American, 154
Scientific journals, 55
Seattle (Indian Chief), 135
Sedatives (see Tranquilizers)
Seeds (also see Germination), 64, 65
Seizures, 96
Self-care/healing, xvi, xxi, xxiii, 4, 15, 16, 29, 71, 79, 96, 122, 140
Self-organization, 4
Self-regulation, 4, 108
Selye, Dr. Hans, 4
Sensitivity (also see Hypersensitivity), 18, 19, 28, 57, 88, 112, 115, 117, 124, 133, 143
Sensory changes, 158
Sepia (cuttlefish), 21, 80, 81, 110, 112, 113, 117
Serum cholesterol (see Cholesterol)
Seward, William, 38, 40
Sexuality, 114, 117, 132, 133
Shadman, Dr. Alonzo, 230
Shakespeare, William, 7, 96, 139
Sharma, R. R., 14
Shellfish (also see Food), 145
Shephard, Dorothy, 231
Shin splints, 174, 179
Shock, 85, 177
Side effects (of drugs), xv, xix, xxii, 29, 66, 75, 83, 93, 95, 98, 101, 107, 109, 111, 116, 121, 128, 141, 142, 143, 147, 155, 157, 175, 181, 186–188, 191–192, 205, 223–224

Silica, 64, 80, 127, 131, 180
Silver, 101, 102
Silver nitrate (see *Argenticum nitricum*)
Similars (see "Law of Similars")
Similimums, 27
Simons, Dr. Marcel, 82
Simpson, O. J., 175
Sinusitis, 131
Skin (also see Acne; Cortisone; Exzema; Injections; Touch), 16, 17, 26, 46, 56, 79, 82, 84, 87, 95, 96, 98, 99, 100, 101, 115, 133, 139, 147, 191, 206
Sleep (also see Dreams; Drowsiness; Insomnia), 97, 103
Sloan-Kettering Institute, 153, 221
Smallpox, 35, 132, 133, 134, 135
Smith, Dr. Trevor, 231, 235
Smoke/Smoking, 115
Snakeroot (see *Actaea racemosa*)
Sneezing (also see Nose), 139, 144
Snowberry (see *Symphoricarpus racemosa*)
Snow-rose (see *Helleborus*)
Society of Homoeopaths, 244, 249
Society of Ultramolecular Medicine, 247
Sodium chloride (see *Natrum mur*)
Sodium sulphate (see *Natrum sulph*)
Sore throat (see Throat)
South Africa, 50
Soviet Union, 15, 50
Spain, 49, 50, 73
Spanish fly (see *Cantharis*)
Spasms, 85, 86, 142
Spiritual practices, xvi, 41
Spock, Dr. Benjamin, 99
Spontaneous remission, 170
Sports/Sports medicine, xx, 85, 173–183
Sports trainers/coaches, 18, 175, 177
Sprains, 178–181
Sprays, 93, 120, 141
Spurge olive (see *Mezereum*)
Sri Lanka, 49
Stapf, Dr. Ernst, 29
Staphylococcus, 127
Staphysagria (stavesacre), 85, 101, 127
Starr, Paul, 37
Star Wars, 15
State Homeopathic Hospital, at Middletown (N.Y.), 197

Statistics, 59, 60, 75, 77, 78, 125, 129, 139, 145, 155
Stavesacre (see *Staphysagria*)
Stebbing, A.R.D., 65
Steffan, William, 65
Steroids, 141, 143, 147, 191
Stiffness (also see Arthritis), 86
Stillbirths (also see Birth), 62, 84
Stinging (also see Bees), 145
Stinging nettle (see *Urtica urens*)
Stomach (also see Abdomen; Digestion; Gastroenteritis), 97, 98, 102, 103, 104, 129, 140
Stowe, Harriet Beecher, 40
Stramonium (thorn-apple), 96
Strange, Michael, 134
Streptococcus/Strep throat (also see Throat), 100, 120, 124, 125
Stress (also see Injuries), xiv, 4, 16, 19, 21, 25, 28, 78, 79, 83, 96, 119, 134, 141, 148, 157, 159, 188, 190, 198, 204, 210
Stress fracture, 174
Styes, 127
Subatomic activity (also see Atoms; Ions; Molecules; Protons), 63
Subotnick, Dr. Steven, 181–182
Succussion (shaking of medicines), 15, 146
Suicide (also see Death), 162, 189, 196
Sulphide of antimony (see *Antimonium crudum*)
Sulphur, 19, 21, 26, 85, 86, 98, 101, 104, 118, 131, 213
Suppression of symptoms (also see Symptoms), xx, xxi, 5, 8, 9, 17, 22, 28, 29, 37, 93, 94, 97, 98, 99, 109, 140, 141, 142, 147, 154, 158–161, 190–192
Surgery/Surgeons, xxiii, 25, 36, 73, 85, 94, 141, 144, 147, 154, 156, 157, 165, 166, 167, 168, 176, 180, 213, 214
Swamps, 120
Sweating (see Perspiration)
Sweden/Swedes, 75
Swelling, 8, 79, 86, 88, 91, 109, 110, 141, 145, 177, 178
Sycotic miasm, 161
Symphoricarpus racemosa (snowberry), 80
Symphytum (comfrey), 180

Syphilinum (exudate from syphilis chancre), 134
Syphilis (also see Venereal diseases), 160

Taft, Dr. Charles, 210
Tandy, Jessica, 42
Tartar emetic (see *Antimonium tart*)
T-cells (also see B-cells; Immune system), 134, 209
Teeth (see Dental problems)
Teething, 22, 57, 96, 97
Telephus, 7
Temperament, 18, 21
Temperature (also see Coldness; Heat), 19
Temporomanibular joint syndrome (TMJ), 214–215
Tennis elbow, 179
Tessier, J. P., 39
Teste, Dr. Alphonse, 87
Tetracycline, 92, 133
Thackeray, William, 41
Thalidomide (also see Birth), 77
Theophylline, 142
Therapeutic double-bind, 198
Thighs (also see Legs), 86
Thirst (also see Drink), 8, 88, 95, 102, 113
Thomas, Lewis, 153, 221
Thompson, Ian, 173
Thorn-apple (see *Stramonium*)
Throat (also see Streptococcus), 9, 86, 120, 122, 123, 124, 125, 127, 143
Thuja (arbor vitae), 134
Thyroid gland, 114, 115, 142, 166, 204
Times (of London), 48, 133, 134
Tissue (also see Muscles; Skin), 86, 120, 121, 149
Toes (also see Legs), 180
Toothache, 211–215
Tooth decay (see Caries)
Toxicity/Toxins (also see Detoxification), 26, 34, 59, 62, 77, 94, 154, 160, 163
Toxicology, 8, 62, 132, 133
Tranquilizers (also see Antidepressants; Emotions), 96, 107, 181
Trauma (see Injury; Stress), 177, 213, 214
Tremors/Trembling, 86, 102
Trichomonas, 111

Tuberculinum (tubercle bacilli), 101, 134
Tuberculosis (also see Lungs), 126
Tumors, 108, 161, 166, 207
Turner, Tina, 3, 29
Twain, Mark, 40
Twitches, 86, 95
Tyler, Margaret, 20, 234
Typhoid fever (also see Epidemics), 57, 125
Typhoidinum (typhoid bacilli), 135
Typology (also see Personality types), 18, 19, 80, 112, 162, 234

Ulcers, 161
Ullman, Dana, 230, 233, 240
Ullman, Dyan, 167
Underactivity (also see Hyperactivity), 23
"Undifferentiated" illness (see "Nonspecific" illness)
University of Glasgow, 59, 146
University of Illinois, 121
University of Iowa, 43
University of Michigan, 39, 43
University of Minnesota, 43
Urination/Urinary tract, 19, 110, 111
Urology, 18
Urtica urens (stinging nettle), 145
U.S. Bureau of Census, xv
U.S. Commission on Education, 43
Uterus (also see Women's health), 83, 84, 108, 110, 116
Vaccines/Vaccination (also see Immunization), 126, 132, 133, 134
Vagina/Vaginitis (also see Women's health), 78, 82, 108, 111, 115, 116, 121, 166
Vakil Prakesh, 235
Valium, 156
Varicellinum (also see Chicken pox), 131
Varicose veins (see Veins)
Variolinum (smallpox exudate), 135
Vegetable charcoal (see *Carbo veg*)
Veins (also see Arteries; Blood; Capillaries; Intravenous fluids), 79, 82, 91, 156, 161
Venereal diseases (also see AIDS; ARC; Chlamydia; Gonorrhea; Herpes; Syphilis), 133, 160
Venom of the bushmaster snake (see

Lachesis)
Venom of the rattlesnake (see *Crotalus horridus*)
Vertigo, 9, 60, 215
Veterinarians, 50, 56, 62, 245, 247
Veterinary schools, 48, 62
Vietnam, 154
Vipera (German viper), 82
Viruses (also see Antiviral agents; Bacteria; Disease; Germs), xiv, xv, xix, 4, 5, 64, 93, 119, 125, 128, 129, 130, 131, 132, 133, 134, 135, 161
Visualization, 219
"Vital force," xx, xxi, 15
Vitamins, 28, 117
Vithoulkas, George, 14, 192, 230
Vomiting, 80, 81, 96, 103
Vulva (also see Women's health), 86

Wald, Dr. Ellen, 124
Waldbolt, George, 207
Warts, 130, 161
Washington, George, 203
Washington Post, 50
Water, 12, 63, 65, 75, 76, 85, 120, 125, 139, 144, 146, 205–211
Watson, Lyall, 189
Weakness (also see Exhaustion), 102, 115, 133, 146, 150, 206, 207, 211
Webster, Daniel, 40
Weight, 101, 133
Weightlifters, 178
Wellness programs, xvi
Wertz, Dorothy, 74
Wertz, Richard, 74
Western Journal of Medicine, 50
West Germany (see Germany)
Wheeler, Dr. Charles, 234
Whitaker, Dr. Julian, 157
White blood cells (also see Blood; Cells), 5, 64, 93, 133
Whitmont, Dr. Edward C., 20, 21, 192, 200
Whooping cough (also see Lungs), 99, 126
Wild hops (see *Bryonia*)
Wild liquorice (see *Sarsaparilla*)
Windflower (see *Pulsatilla*)
Witch hazel (see *Hamamelis*)
Women physicians, 41, 45
Women's health (also see Birth; Breastfeeding; Breasts; Cervix; Gynecology; Lactation; Menopause; Menstruation; Ovaries; Postpartum period; Pregnancy; Premenstrual syndrome; Reproductive system; Uterus; Vagina; Vulva), xx, 107–118
Women's medical schools, 41
Wood, Matthew, 234
World Health Forum, 49
World Health Organization (WHO), 49, 75, 133, 134
World War II, 59

Yeast (also see *Candida albicans*), 65, 121
Yeats, William Butler, 41
Yellow fever (also see Epidemics), 43, 57, 125, 126
Yellow jasmine (see *Gelsemium*)
Yiamouyiannis, Dr. John, 206, 207
Yoga, 15
Yogurt (also see Food), 103

Zand, Dr. Janet, 179, 180
Zaren, Ananda, 78, 81, 82, 83
Zellerbach, Merla, 150
Zinc, 96, 101, 178

About the Author

Dana Ullman received his masters in public health from U.C. Berkeley. He coauthored (with Stephen Cummings) *Everybody's Guide to Homeopathic Medicines*, which is one of the most popular guidebooks to using homeopathic medicines. This book won the *Medical Self-Care* "Book Award" and has been translated into five languages. Dana is the founder and President of the Foundation for Homeopathic Education and Research, is an elected Board member of the National Center for Homeopathy, and directs Homeopathic Educational Services, a primary distributor of homeopathic books, tapes, and medicine kits in the United States.

Dana Ullman has edited *Monograph on Homeopathic Research* (volumes I and II) and has served as publisher of seven books in homeopathy by other authors. He has also written over 50 published articles in a variety of respected publications, including *Western Journal of Medicine, Social Policy, Medical Self-Care, New Age, California Living* (the Sunday supplement magazine to the *San Francisco Chronicle* and *San Francisco Examiner*), *Mother Earth News*, as well as numerous alternative health care and homeopathic journals and newsletters.

Dana Ullman has been particularly effective in working with major institutions and getting them to change their attitudes and policies towards natural health care. He has organized successful conferences that were sponsored or co-sponsored by the federal Department of Health & Human Services, U.C. Berkeley School of Public Health, and innumerable community organizations. He authored the San Francisco Foundation's *Health Report*, which changed the funding priorities of this major philanthropic institution. In another health policy area, he consulted on a research project sponsored by the California medical board which recommended many of his proposals.

Dana Ullman has made some of the most significant contributions enabling homeopathic medicine and natural health care gain the increasing recognition and popularity they are presently experiencing. Besides acting as an advocate for the new health movement, Dana has helped provide some essential critique of this movement in order to deepen its influence on health care and broaden its impact on society at large.